Type 2 Diabetes Cookbook

60 Healthy And Quick Recipes For Appetizers, Salads And Low Carb Breads To Live A More Peaceful And Serene Life With A Daily Diet Plan

© Copyright 2021 by **Elizabeth Stuckey**

Table of Contents

Preface

The following indications have an EXCLUSIVE informative purpose and are not intended to replace the opinion of professional figures such as doctors, nutritionists or dieticians, whose intervention is necessary for the prescription and composition of PERSONALIZED food therapies.

Chapter 1 - Type 2 Diabetes Mellitus

Diabetes Mellitus Type 2 is a disease that affects glucose metabolism; if left untreated, this form of diabetes also affects the state of health, lowering the quality and life expectancy of the patient.

In Diabetes Mellitus Type 2, glucose, once absorbed from the intestinal tract and poured into the circulatory stream - due to an alteration of the hormonal vehicle (insulin) or a malfunction of peripheral tyrosine kinase receptors that do not capture it effectively enough - remains in the circulation causing a series of negative metabolic reactions (NB. The nervous tissue is the only insulin-independent).

Diabetes Mellitus Type 2 is a disorder that includes many facets, but what is common to ALL clinical pictures is a situation of hyperglycemia (>110 mg/dl), possibly accompanied by hyper-insulinemia and hyperlipidemia (VLDL - hypertriglyceridemia); Obviously, this frequently leads to overweight, aggravation of hypertension, glycation of plasma proteins, pro-oxidation of APO-protein B and consequent REDUCTION of the ability to bind to peripheral receptors (LDL hypercholesterolemia), increased risk of atherosclerosis, retinopathy, neuropathy, nephropathy and diabetic foot.

Causes and Treatment

Diabetes Mellitus Type 2 has several etiological causes; the most common are related to lifestyle: poor diet and abuse of carbohydrates, excess of fat mass, lack of muscle mass, sedentariness; others are genetic, such as structural alteration of insulin or peripheral receptors. Certainly, whatever the causes, the most effective therapy for Diabetes Mellitus

Type 2 consists of:

- Reducing overweight/obesity
- Reduction of excess carbohydrates and restoration of nutritional balance
- Motor therapy
- Pharmacological therapy
- Compensation of other dysmetabolisms.

Diet for Diabetes Mellitus Type 2

The diet for Diabetes Mellitus Type 2 is almost always constituted by a low-calorie regimen (for weight loss) and, if not hypoglucidic, that provides the least amount of carbohydrates possible while maintaining a certain nutritional balance; the diet for Diabetes Mellitus Type 2 CANNOT be separated from the beginning of a motor therapy.

The basic principles of the diet for Diabetes Mellitus Type 2 are:

- Hypocaloricity (if necessary)

- Reduction of the overall glycemic load
- Reduction of the glycemic load of meals
- Reduction of the glycemic index of meals

Simple carbohydrate intake exclusively represented by fructose naturally present in vegetables or lactose naturally present in milk and dairy products (if possible, simple CHOs should remain around 10-12% of total calories).

Which, from a practical standpoint, translates into:

- Choosing fibre-rich foods and drastically eliminating/reducing refined foods
- Abolition of sweets, sweet carbonated drinks, fruit juices, beer and baked goods
- Reduction of fruit that is too sweet and elimination of preserved fruit (candied, syrupy, jams (questionable), dehydrated etc.)
- Increase, as much as possible, foods containing antioxidants (vegetables, fruits NOT too sugary).

Useful supplements

There are no fundamental supplements to the treatment/diet for Diabetes Mellitus Type 2 (drugs are NOT supplements); however, it is obvious that a well-considered supplementation based on antioxidants (to try to improve the oxidative stress on lipoproteins) and, in the case of a strongly hypocaloric diet, a supplement of fibre (possibly viscous that improve the glycemic index of the meal and increase the sense of satiety) could be useful in improving the impact of nutritional treatment.

Chapter 2 – Recipes for Diabetics and Standards for a Healthy Diet

General Dietary Recommendations

- Reduce consumption of simple sugars.
- Reduce consumption of saturated fats.
- Increase fiber consumption.
- Never skip breakfast.
- Eat complete meals (carbohydrates + protein + vegetables + fruit) at lunch and dinner.
- Avoid prolonged periods of fasting.
- Share equally, in the 3 main meals, the total amount of complex carbohydrates (bread, pasta, rice, rusks).

In following the indications it should be however considered that, in order to obtain a correct and balanced nutrition which supplies the body with all the nutrients it needs, it is necessary to assume the right quantity (portion) of food and to respect the frequency with which some foods must be consumed, daily or weekly, within a personalized food scheme.

The daily nutrition must respect the energy balance of each person and the energy introduced must be equal to the one spent in order not to increase the risk of overweight, obesity as well as malnutrition.

Food not allowed

- White sugar and brown sugar or fructose to sweeten beverages, substituting sweetener if necessary.
- Jam and honey.
- Sweets such as cakes, pastries, cookies, shortbread, jellies, puddings, candies.
- Fruit in syrup, candied fruit, fruit mustard.
- Sugary drinks such as cola, tonic water, iced tea, as well as fruit juices, because they naturally contain sugar even if they are labeled "no added sugar".
- Sauces containing sugar such as ketchup.
- Fatty condiments such as butter, lard, margarine.
- Sausages.
- Spirits.

Food allowed in moderation

It is important to respect the quantities indicated in the diet and limit to occasional consumption the sugariest fruits (grapes, bananas, figs, persimmons, tangerines).

- Fruits as they naturally contain sugar (fructose).
- Sweetener.
- Dietary bakery products for diabetics, remembering that although sugar-free they are not low-calorie, but have a caloric value almost equal to traditional analogues.
- Red wine (about half glass per meal).
- Salt. It is a good rule to reduce the amount of salt added to food during and after cooking and to limit the consumption of foods which naturally contain high quantities of salt (canned or pickled foods, meat cubes and extracts, soy sauces).
- Chestnuts are not a fruit and potatoes and corn are not a vegetable.

These foods are important sources of starch therefore they are real substitutes of bread, pasta and rice.

Therefore they can be occasionally consumed as a substitute of the first course.

- Legumes (chickpeas, beans, peas, broad beans, etc.) should be limited, as they contain carbohydrates and therefore raise blood sugar; however they are also an important source of vegetable proteins (therefore they can be considered as real and proper second courses).

It is advisable to consume them in association with cereals (1 or 2 times a week) therefore making unique dishes.

Allowed and recommended foods

- Raw and cooked vegetables to be consumed in generous portions.
- Fish (fresh or frozen) no less than two to three times a week.
- Complex carbohydrates (bread, pasta, rice, toast) and whole grains.
- Olive oil, added raw and in moderation.
- Cheese to be consumed a couple of times a week, as an alternative to the second course.
- You can take a couple of teaspoons (15 gr) of grated Grana Padano D.O.P. per day.
- Leaner sliced meats (cooked ham, raw ham, bresaola, speck, roast turkey and chicken) depriving them of visible fat.

- Red and white meat (from lean cuts and without visible fat). Skinless poultry.
- Skimmed or semi-skimmed milk and yogurt.
- Water, at least 1.5 litres per day (preferably low-mineral water).

Behavioral Rules

In case of overweight or obesity it is recommended the reduction of weight and of the "waistline", that is the abdominal circumference, indicator of the amount of fat deposited at visceral level.

Waist circumference values above 94 cm in men and 80 cm in women are associated with a "moderate" cardiovascular risk, values above 102 cm in men and 88 cm in women are associated with a "high risk". Returning to a normal weight allows not only to reduce blood glucose levels, but also to reduce other cardiovascular risk factors (such as hypertension, hypercholesterolemia, hypertriglyceridemia).

- Make your lifestyle more active (give up being sedentary! Walk, bike, or park far to work; if you can, avoid using the elevator and walk the stairs).
- Practice physical activity at least three times a week both aerobic and muscle strengthening (anaerobic).

Constant physical activity has beneficial effects on people with diabetes, as well as being essential to eliminate excess fat and lose weight properly.

Read product labels, especially to ascertain their sugar content. Pay attention to the use of "sugar-free" products as they are often rich in fat and consequently high in calories.

Practical Tips

The patient with diabetes mellitus type 2 should include in his diet

- a breakfast consisting of: a cup of semi-skimmed milk or a pot of low-fat yogurt + rusks or bread or cereals or dry cookies plus a medium-sized fruit (about 150 g), to be eaten preferably with the skin, well washed.

- at lunch and dinner complete meals, consisting of: bread, pasta or rice (preferably cooked "al dente", using in about 50% of cases whole grains) plus main course (meat or fish or cheese or sliced meats or eggs or legumes) plus vegetables plus a fruit. Those who do not want to eat first and second course, can make unique dishes based on carbohydrates and proteins such as pasta with tuna, rice and pasta with legumes, pasta with mozzarella and tomato, roast beef sandwich, always accompanied by vegetables and a fruit.
- possible snacks between meals or in the late evening, if you are accustomed to eat dinner early (before 20), based on fresh fruit, low-fat yogurt with a tablespoon of cereals without sugar, or a glass of milk or a few flakes of Parmigiano cheese (10-15 g) with a couple of rusks.

Warnings

The dietary advices provided are purely indicative and must not be considered a substitute for the indications of the doctor, as some patients may require dietary adaptations based on their individual clinical situation.

The ideal diet is one that prefers legumes, fruits, vegetables and whole grains.

Legumes

One of the foods that should never be missing on the table of those who suffer from diabetes (but not only), are legumes. It is, in fact, a super food able to bring numerous benefits to our body.

Legumes, thanks to the high content of soluble fibre, help to keep under control the levels of glucose in the blood.

So, bringing lentils, peas, chickpeas and beans to the table two-three times a week is, without a doubt, a healthy choice. In addition, always the presence of fibre increases the sense of satiety.

All this helps to avoid hunger attacks and various binges responsible for weight gain.

Fruits and vegetables should never be missing in a varied and balanced diet.

Vegetables also play an important role in the diet of diabetics as they help to control the absorption of sugar in the blood.

The ideal is to consume five portions of vegetables a day, varying as much as possible "color" and type.

As for vegetables, they should never be missing in every meal (both at lunch and dinner).

Fruits and vegetables are beneficial for those who suffer from diabetes. Fibre keeps glucose values under control, increases the level of satiety and helps to return to a healthy weight, specifies the expert.

Those who are overweight or obese are more likely to suffer from diabetes.

Whole grain bread and pasta

Who suffers from diabetes should prefer complex carbohydrates, contained in cereals, preferably whole grain.

Green light to pasta or brown rice seasoned with vegetables and legumes, sprinkled with a drizzle of raw evo oil.

First courses based on whole grains, enriched with vegetable sauces, provide an excellent intake of fibre, with beneficial effects on health (glucose and fat under control, greater satiety).

The Mediterranean diet (rich in fruits, vegetables, fish and whole grains) is therefore also suitable for the diet of diabetics.

Not only whole-grain pasta, bread and rice: to vary the diet, you can alternate satisfying pasta dishes to tasty one-dish meals based on cereals and legumes such as, for example, kamut and lentils or, again, couscous of spelt, peas and vegetables.

Attention to drink

Not only food, if you need to keep blood sugar under control you must also pay attention to what you drink.

For example, those who suffer from diabetes should avoid the consumption of sugary drinks, such as: cola, orangeade, sodas, fruit juices and various cocktails.

These are real "sugar bombs" that rapidly raise blood sugar levels.

"In addition, sugary drinks bring the so-called "empty" calories, that is, devoid of nutrition."

Also beware of hidden, well-disguised sugar: contained, for example, in fruit in syrup and sweet snacks.

Prefer foods with low energy density

Among the foods to avoid, to ward off blood sugar spikes, are all those foods with high caloric density.

"Foods that are high in fat and simple sugars but low in water generally provide a lot of energy in a small volume.

These are the energy-dense foods like a slice of chocolate cake or a sandwich with mayonnaise, or even sausages."

Foods rich in water and fibre such as fruits, vegetables and whole grains, on the other hand, provide few calories in a large volume and are defined as low energy density.

The stomach is "deceived" by the volume of food and, therefore, foods or preparations that have a low energy density have a greater satiating power.

An example: first courses based on whole grains, legumes and vegetables.

A glass of wine a day

Alcohol, in case one suffers from diabetes or if one is overweight, should be avoided.

In case, once in a while, one wants to indulge in a glass of wine, it is appropriate to keep an eye on the quantity allowed.

A moderate intake of alcohol, up to 10 grams/day for women (one serving) and 20 grams/day for men (two servings), is acceptable.

However, diabetics should avoid drinks such as hard liquor cocktails altogether.

The same goes for non-alcoholic mixes, which are very rich in simple sugars and empty calories.

Lots of fibre

pasta al dente, cold potatoes: here are the practical suggestions for the diet of those who have problems with insulin.

Strict restrictions in the diet of those with type 2 diabetes, the most common?

That era is gone, because some tricks allow you to eat in a tasty way trying to keep blood sugar at bay. Or by respecting certain dietary regimens or by learning some simple rules to cook in a healthier way.

There are also some clichés to dismantle. Contrary to popular belief, the basis for a balanced diet in diabetics is also carbohydrate and fibre-rich foods such as fruits and vegetables.

Diabetes and hypertension.

In short, the plate of spaghetti is welcome. Today, diabetes is no longer considered, as it was a few years ago, a kind of allergy to sugar.

Carbohydrates are not only allowed, but recommended, because they are necessary for the body.

So how should the diet be for those who have problems with insulin?

I try to summarize a simple message for the choices at the table in type 2 diabetes: you can eat anything, but you can't eat a lot.

A 5-10% weight loss is enough to optimize disease control, but also to halve the risk of becoming diabetic in an overweight or obese person.

The problem is growing.

According to the latest data, Italians with type 2 diabetes (non-autoimmune) are over 3.5 million and in 2030 will be, according to estimates, over 5 million.

This is a chronic disease, characterized by the presence of high levels of glucose in the blood (hyperglycemia) and due to an altered amount or activity of insulin (the hormone, produced by the pancreas, which allows glucose to enter the cells and its subsequent use as an energy source).

To cope with it, you need to change your eating habits.

Throughout life.

But it must be experienced as a change, not as a deprivation.

Often totally eliminating certain foods can be more dangerous than indulging in them in a reasoned way.

Here are some tips on proper nutrition for diabetics.

With one caveat: it is advisable to define a personalized diet plan with a specialist.

Tricks for lowering the glycemic index.

It is useful for a diabetic to learn to distinguish foods based on the glycemic index.

This parameter indicates how quickly the glucose in food is absorbed by the blood.

When we eat a food rich in carbohydrates, glucose levels in the bloodstream gradually increase as starches and sugars are digested and assimilated.

The speed of these processes changes according to the food and the type of nutrients it contains, the amount of fibre present and the composition of other foods already present in the stomach and intestine.

The glycemic index is mainly related to foods high in carbohydrates, whereas those rich in fat or proteins do not have an immediate effect on blood sugar levels (glycemia), but determine a delayed and prolonged increase.

The glycemic index is influenced by the composition of foods, but also by cooking methods.

They tend to reduce it, for example, the partial boiling (spaghetti al dente and not cooked are good in every sense) or the cooling of cooked foods, such as boiled potatoes.

Also the presence of foods with soluble fibres, capable of absorbing high quantities of water, forming in the intestine a sort of gel, helps to lower the glycemic index.

But what happens, instead, if you overdo with foods with high glycemic index?

A rapid rise in blood sugar levels causes the pancreas to secrete large amounts of insulin.

And insulin causes a rapid utilization of glucose by the tissues, so that two-three hours after the meal, hypoglycemia is determined, resulting in a feeling of hunger and a certain discomfort. If you ingest more carbohydrates to cope with hunger, you stimulate a new secretion of insulin and you enter a vicious circle.

This is not the only danger.

Often the body doesn't use all the glucose, so it is converted into fat tissue.

Unused fat reserves accumulate and generate overweight.

Not all scholars, however, evaluate the usefulness of the glycemic index in the same way.

The American Diabetes Association (ADA) has even questioned its clinical usefulness, recommending that attention be paid more to the quantity of food than to the source of carbohydrates.

A well-balanced diet is the essential cure for diabetes.

Following a controlled and healthy diet serves above all to keep the blood sugar level under control through a correct dietary intake of all nutrients necessary for the health of the body.

An excessive diet compared to the real needs increases the need for insulin, forcing the pancreas to a super-activity; all this can result in an insufficient production of insulin to cope with the demands generated by an unbalanced and inadequate diet.

In these cases, reaching and maintaining the ideal weight with an appropriate diet is often sufficient to obtain a good control of diabetes itself.

Caloric Supply

The ideal diabetic diet is not at all complex or restrictive.

The diabetic patient needs a daily caloric intake equal to that of the non-diabetic subject, in relation to: physical constitution, sex, age, height, work activity, etc., having as objective the achievement and maintenance of the ideal body weight.

If there is no need to achieve rapid weight loss, with a reduction of about 900 calories per day you can achieve a weight loss of about 3 kg per month, which can be further increased with the usual daily practice of moderate physical activity (walking or cycling flat, walking the dog, do not use elevators, walk to work, etc.).

The distribution of calories among foods

In the daily diet must be carefully evaluated the intake of simple sugars with rapid absorption (glucose and sucrose) giving preference to complex sugars with slow absorption (starch).

The total daily intake of carbohydrates should not exceed 50-55% of total calories, provided that at least 80% of it is starch and the remaining 20% is non-insulin dependent sugars and fibre.

Fibres must be taken in high quantities, especially the water-soluble ones, capable of slowing down the intestinal absorption of carbohydrates and cholesterol.

Proteins must make up about 15%-20% of total calories and at least one third must be animal proteins, rich in essential amino acids.

The remaining calories (25%-30%) must be provided by fats, possibly of vegetable origin, with a high content of polyunsaturated fatty acids, useful in the prevention of cardiovascular diseases.

The intake of vitamins and minerals must also be adequate.

The exchange between foods and equivalents

Each food can be substituted by another one or by some others, provided they belong to the same group; it is also possible the substitution between foods belonging to different groups, provided they have a similar content of nutrients.

In the diabetic's diet, the system of food exchange allows to plan meals according to taste.

One way to exchange foods while maintaining the caloric intake is to group them according to their sugar content.

Three main carbohydrate amounts (equivalents) were arbitrarily chosen:

- Milk equivalent (for milk): 10gr of carbohydrates

- Fruit equivalent (for fruit): 10gr of carbohydrates

- Bread equivalent (for cereals and legumes): 25gr of carbohydrates

Within the various groups, the weight of various foods providing the same amount of carbohydrates was determined.

In each group of equivalents all the foods belonging to it can be substituted with each other because they all have the same value.

For example are equivalent milk 200ml of low fat milk and a pot of natural yogurt; are equivalent fruits 100gr of pear, 130gr of peach and 80gr of grape; are equivalent bread 50gr of white bread, 100gr of cooked spaghetti and 70gr of pizza.

Meat and Protein Equivalent

For meat and cheese the equivalence is about proteins and fats.

A lean meat equivalent (ex. sole) corresponds to 100gr of edible part and can be substituted by 80gr of semi-fat meat (ex. sirloin of beef) or by 60gr of fat meat (ex. salami) or by 60gr of cheese (ex. ricotta or parmesan).

Appetizers

Vegan Fish Croquettes

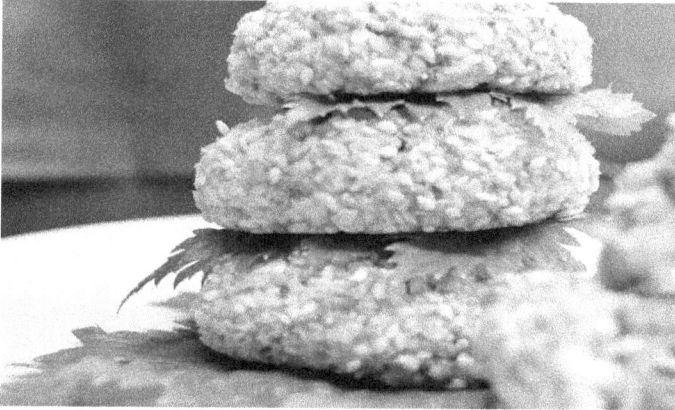

Recipe ID card

~ 97 Kcal Calories per serving
~ Difficulty quite easy
~ Serves 3
~ Preparation 20 minutes
~ Average cost
~ 20 minutes for preparation; 15 minutes for cooking

Ingredients for 10-12 meatballs

~ 10 g breadcrumbs
~ 8 g of brewer's yeast flakes
~ Dehydrated food: 20 g of daikon
~ 1 tablespoon of extra virgin olive oil
~ pepper
~ salt
~ Ready-to-boil food: 140 g chickpeas
~ 10 g of wakame seaweed
~ 100 g of tofu

To coat

~ 30 g of poppy seeds
~ 2 tbsp extra virgin olive oil
~ 30 g of sesame seeds

Material Required

~ Blender
~ Colander
~ Bowls
~ Cutting board
~ Spoons

Preparation

Gather wakame seaweed in a bowl and cover with cold water to rehydrate: 5 minutes is enough.

Meanwhile, also soak the dried daikon in cold water for 5 minutes.

Squeeze the seaweed and daikon out of the soaking water and combine the ingredients in the glass of a blender.

Add the hemp seed tofu, boiled chickpeas, brewer's yeast flakes, a tablespoon of oil, and salt and pepper to taste.

Check the consistency of the mixture: if it is too soft, add as much bread crumbs as needed until the desired creaminess is achieved.

Preheat oven to 180°C.

Take a spoonful of the mixture and roll it in the sesame seeds. Crush the mixture between your hands to form croquettes: you will obtain 10-12 croquettes.

Gradually place the croquettes on an oven tray, add a couple of tablespoons of oil and bake at 180°C for 15 minutes or until golden brown.

Serve the croquettes still very hot, with mustard sauce or vegan mayonnaise.

Caponata Light

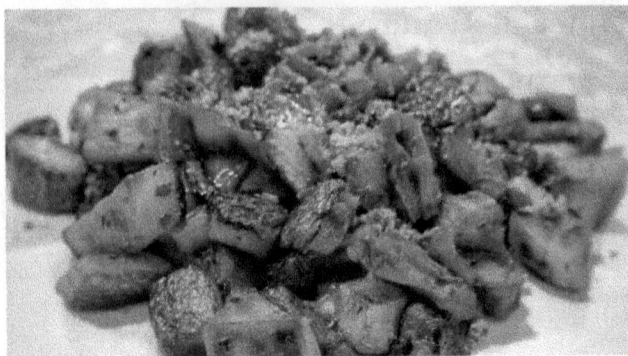

Recipe ID card

- ~ 52 Kcal Calorie per porzione
- ~ Difficoltà molto facile
- ~ Dosi per 4 persone
- ~ Preparazione 35 minuti
- ~ Costo medio
- ~ Nota 20 minuti di cottura + il tempo di preparazione delle verdure (15 minuti)

Ingredients

- ~ 1 tuft of basil
- ~ 300 g of celery
- ~ 1 pinch of coarse salt
- ~ 300 g of coppery tomatoes
- ~ 30 g of pine nuts
- ~ a pinch of pepper
- ~ 75 g of black olives
- ~ 2 tablespoons of extra virgin olive oil
- ~ 700 g of eggplants
- ~ 40 g of capers
- ~ 1 pinch of salt

Material Required

- ~ Plates
- ~ Bowls
- ~ Food cutting board
- ~ Ceramic knife
- ~ Pasta strainer
- ~ Casserole
- ~ Large frying pan with lid

Preparation

Clean the eggplants: wash them well, remove the stalk, cut them into slices about 1.5 cm thick and cut them into cubes. Place the diced eggplants on a colander: add a pinch of coarse salt and let them drain: in this way, the eggplants will lose the excess water and, with it, also the typical bitter aftertaste. Let the eggplants drain for at least one hour.

In the meantime, peel the tomatoes. To facilitate the operation, cut the end opposite the stem with a cross and plunge the tomatoes into boiling water for about ten seconds. Remove the tomatoes from the water and peel them. Cut them into small pieces and pour them into a saucepan.

Toast the pine nuts and add them to the tomatoes.

Desalt the capers, cut the olives into small pieces and add them to the tomato. Season with salt and pepper to taste.

Clean the celery and cut it into small pieces. Add the celery to the sauce, season with salt and pepper and add a drizzle of extra virgin olive oil. Cook everything on a low heat for 20-30 minutes.

Rinse the eggplants well, dry them and brown them in a large pan, avoiding adding too much oil. Keep a lively flame.

Finish cooking the eggplant by adding the tomato sauce.

Let the eggplant cool and serve with a few leaves of fresh basil.

Octopus Carpaccio

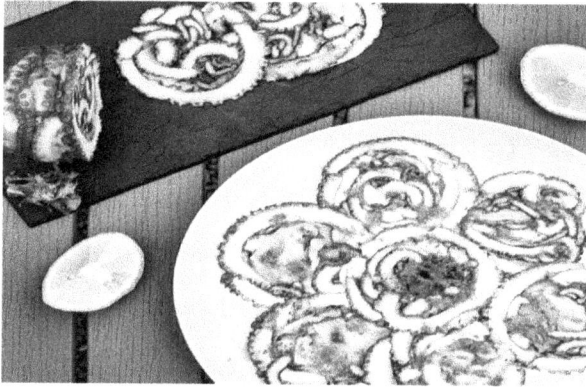

Recipe ID card

- ~ 81 Kcal calories per serving
- ~ Easy difficulty
- ~ Serves 4
- ~ Preparation 35 minutes
- ~ Average cost
- ~ 20 minutes for cooking octopus + 15 minutes for preparation; 3 hours cooling time

Ingredients

- ~ 1 Kg of octopus
- ~ Untreated lemon juice
- ~ 2 spoons of extra virgin olive oil
- ~ 1 tuft of parsley
- ~ salt
- ~ pepper
- ~ 100 g of black olives
- ~ 30 g of capers

Material Required

- ~ Casserole
- ~ Plastic bottle
- ~ Knife
- ~ Tray or dish to collect the liquid
- ~ Cutting board
- ~ Serving dish
- ~ Meat tenderizer or other weight (e.g. glass jar filled with water)

Preparation

Clean the Octopus.

Boil the octopus, calculating 18-20 minutes of cooking time per kilo of shellfish. Turn off the heat and let the octopus cool in its cooking water to soften the flesh.

If you wish, you can remove the skin from the octopus using a small knife or paper towels.

Cut the octopus into pieces, following the tentacles.

Cut a plastic bottle in half, horizontally.

Place the pieces of octopus in the bottom of the bottle, pressing as much as possible in order to remove excess liquid.

Place the half bottle with the octopus in a plate and place a weight on it (e.g. meat pounder or a glass jar full of water). The weight will exert the right pressure on the octopus so that the carpaccio, once sliced, remains compact and does not crumble. In order to remove any excess liquid, turn the bottle with the octopus upside down on the sink. After having removed the liquid, place the weight again.

Place the bottle in the refrigerator, covering it with a nylon bag.

After 2-3 hours, the octopus will have congealed and created a jelly in the empty spaces.

Gently remove the octopus from the bottle, cutting the plastic (if necessary): the result will be a compact cylinder of octopus.

Now cut the octopus carpaccio into thin slices and arrange them on a plate. Make a citronette sauce by emulsifying oil, lemon, salt and pepper. Sprinkle the octopus with the sauce and serve with plenty of parsley, black olives and capers.

Tuna Carpaccio

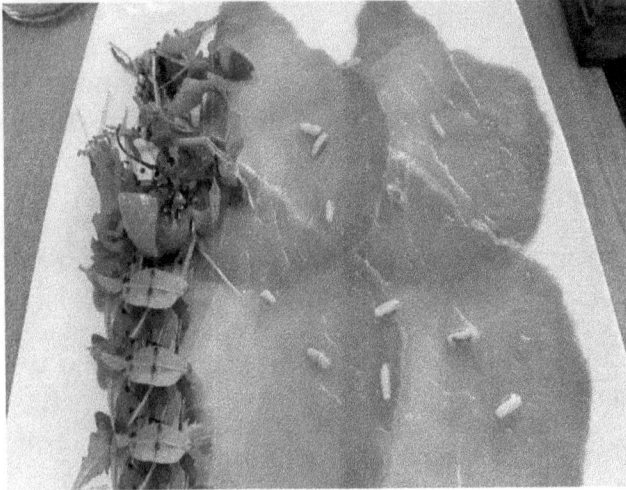

Recipe ID card

~ 146 Kcal calories per serving
~ Easy difficulty
~ Serves 2
~ Preparation 15 minutes
~ Average cost
~ 15 minutes for preparation; 1 hour rest for marinating

Ingredients

For the Carpaccio

~ 200 g of thin slices of fresh tuna fish
~ 50 g of rocket
~ 20 g of sesame seeds

For the marinade

~ fennel
~ 1 sprig of thyme
~ 1 tablespoon of pink pepper
~ 2 tablespoons of extra virgin olive oil
~ Juice and zest of untreated lemon
~ Juice and zest of lime
~ 1 pinch of salt

Material Required

~ Serving dish
~ Colander
~ Frying pan
~ Cutting board
~ Knife
~ Grater or lemon line

Preparation

Wash the lemon and lime thoroughly. Grate the zest and squeeze the juice.

Place the tuna slices on a plate, pour in the lemon and lime juice. Add 1 tablespoon of mild olive oil. Flavor with citrus zest, pink peppercorns, thyme and fennel. Salt to taste.

Cover with a sheet of plastic wrap and let macerate for one hour.

Now remove the tuna from the maceration and arrange the dish. Place a few rocket leaves on the bottom of the plate and dress with a dash of oil, lemon juice and a pinch of salt.

Then lay the tuna carpaccio on top of the rocket, seasoning with one or two spoonfuls of marinade.

Toast the sesame seeds and sprinkle them on top of the tuna carpaccio.

Decorate with lemon zest and herbs. Serve immediately.

Savoury Pie with Spinach

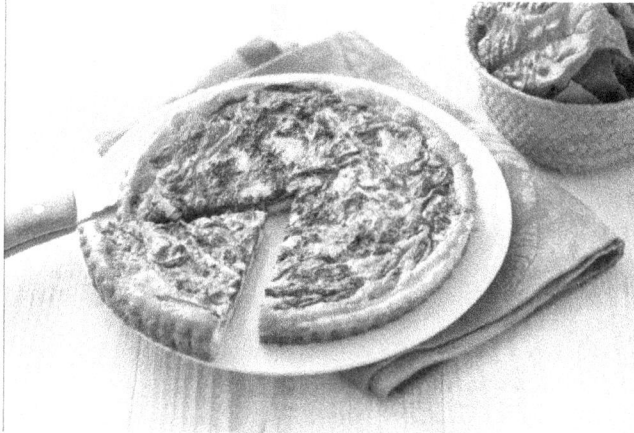

Recipe ID card

- ~ Difficulty quite easy
- ~ Serves 8
- ~ Preparation 30 minutes
- ~ Low cost
- ~ 30 minutes to prepare; 15 minutes to cook spinach; 40 minutes to bake savoury pie

Ingredients

For the vegan pastry

- ~ Half a teaspoon of instant yeast
- ~ 6 g of salt
- ~ 30 ml of water
- ~ 45 ml of extra virgin olive oil
- ~ 75 g of soy yogurt
- ~ 225 g of whole wheat flour

To brush

- ~ soy milk
- ~ 1 pinch of turmeric

For the filling

- ~ 1 teaspoon of turmeric
- ~ 100 g of vegetable ricotta or tofu
- ~ 50 g of vegetable cream
- ~ 50 g of grated Vegan cheese
- ~ pepper

- ~ salt
- ~ 3 tablespoons of extra virgin olive oil
- ~ 1 clove of garlic
- ~ Steamed food: 450 g of spinach

Material Required

- ~ Bowls
- ~ Food weighing scales
- ~ Casserole for steaming
- ~ Ceramic baking dish with a diameter of 24 cm
- ~ Chopping board
- ~ Knife
- ~ Paintbrush
- ~ Baking paper
- ~ Matter
- ~ Spoons
- ~ Transparent film
- ~ Sieve

Preparation

Start the recipe by preparing the dough. In a bowl, combine the organic whole-wheat flour and add the salt and sieved instant yeast. In the center, add the extra virgin olive oil, cold water and unsweetened soy yogurt. Mix all the ingredients, first with a wooden spoon, then by hand, until you get a soft and elastic ball. Wrap the dough in a sheet of plastic wrap and let rest for half an hour.

Meanwhile, prepare the spinach. Wash the spinach leaves, rinse them and steam them until soft. Let the spinach cool, remove it from the pot and squeeze it to remove the vegetation water. Chop the spinach with a knife or a half-moon until chopped. Combine the spinach in a saucepan, add the oil, salt and pepper. If desired, add a clove of garlic for flavor. Let the spinach season on a gentle-moderate flame for 10 minutes. Turn off the flame and allow to cool.

Line a low-sided ceramic baking dish with baking paper.

Divide the whole-wheat brisè pastry into two parts, one slightly larger than the other. Roll out the larger ball with a rolling pin to obtain a disc slightly larger than the size of the pan, a few millimetres thick. Line the baking pan with the disc obtained: the dough should come out from the edges of the pan.

Prepare the second disk following the same procedure, and set aside: the second disk will serve as a cover for the savoury pie. Cover with plastic wrap to prevent the dough from drying out.

Devote time to preparing the filling. Combine the spinach in a bowl, add the vegan grated cheese and vegetable cream. If necessary, adjust the salt.

Fill the whole wheat pastry shell with the spinach filling.

Make small grooves in the filling, then fill the holes with some of the vegetable ricotta. Alternatively, you can use blended tofu.

Mix the remaining ricotta with a teaspoon of turmeric: you will get a yellow cream that will simulate the "yolk" effect. Finish filling the grooves with the yellow-colored ricotta.

Cover with the second disk and seal the edges by pinching the two parts with your hands. If desired, decorate the surface with a whole wheat pastry columbine.

Mix the soy milk with a pinch of turmeric. Brush the surface of the erbazzone with the soy milk and turmeric solution.

Bake the savoury pie in a preheated oven at 180°C for about 40 minutes.

Remove from the oven, leave to cool and serve.

Oven Stuffed Pumpkin Flowers

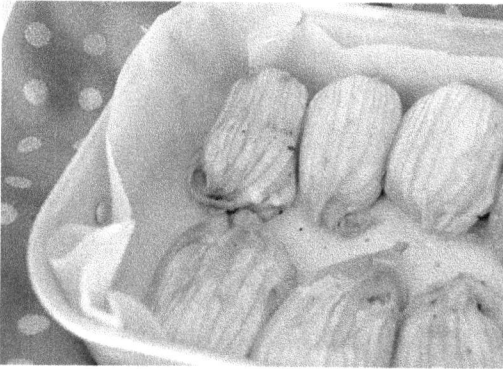

Recipe ID card

- ~ 107 Kcal calories per serving
- ~ Easy difficulty
- ~ Serves 4
- ~ Preparation 35 minutes
- ~ Low cost
- ~ 15 minutes preparation + 15-20 minutes cooking time

Ingredients

For the zucchini flowers

- ~ about ten zucchini flowers
- ~ a handful of rocket
- ~ pepper
- ~ salt
- ~ 1 tablespoon of extra virgin olive oil
- ~ 20 g of sesame seeds
- ~ 200 g of zucchini
- ~ 100 g of Greek yogurt
- ~ 100 g of fresh ricotta

For brushing

- ~ 40 g (1 medium) egg white
- ~ enough sesame seeds
- ~ a pinch of salt
- ~ a pinch of pepper

Material Required

- ~ Pocket knife
- ~ Blotting paper
- ~ Bowl
- ~ Frying pan
- ~ Wooden ladle
- ~ Immersion mixer
- ~ Baking tray
- ~ Sac à poche (optional)
- ~ Scissors

Preparation

Wash the zucchini, remove the ends and cut them into small pieces: sauté them in a pan for about ten minutes with a drizzle of oil, salt and pepper.

Clean squash blossoms by gently opening them with hands: remove central pistil and wash with fresh water. Dab the zucchini flowers with paper towels or a soft cloth.

In the meantime, the zucchini will have softened. Pour the zucchini into an immersion blender and blend until creamy.

In a bowl, pour the ricotta, Greek yogurt (0% fat), zucchini puree, sesame seeds and chopped arugula. Season to taste with salt and pepper.

Pour the mixture into a sac à poche and fill the squash blossoms.

Peel the egg, taking care to separate the yolk from the white. Lightly beat the egg white with a fork and brush the surface of all the zucchini flowers: this way, the zucchini flowers will remain crispy.

Spread some of the ricotta mixture on the baking tray and place the stuffed zucchini flowers on top. Sprinkle with a few sesame seeds.

Bake the pan at 350°F for about 15-20 minutes, until the surface is golden brown.

Serve the stuffed squash blossoms steaming, perhaps accompanying with some fresh arugula.

Vegetable cheese with pea flour

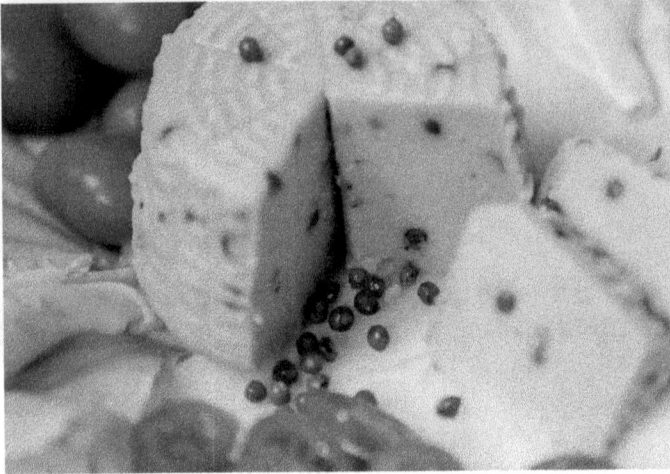

Recipe ID card

~ 161 Kcal calories per serving
~ Easy difficulty
~ Serves 4
~ Preparation 15 minutes
~ Low cost
~ 15 minutes + cooling time

Ingredients

~ 50 g of pea flour
~ 125 g of soy yogurt
~ 2 tablespoons of extra virgin olive oil
~ 70 ml of soy milk
~ 1 pinch of salt
~ 1 tablespoon of pink pepper berries

Material Required

~ Bowl
~ Small casserole
~ Whisk
~ Wooden spoon

Preparation

In a small saucepan, mix the pea flour with a pinch of salt and the pink peppercorns.

Pour in the center the plain soy yogurt, oil, and drizzle in the soy milk (unsweetened). Stir until you have a thick batter.

Place the saucepan on the heat and stir continuously, keeping a gentle-to-moderate flame, until the mixture begins to thicken.

Allow about 2 minutes from the time of boiling, then pour the mixture (which will appear very thick and sticky) into a cheese mold.

Flatten the veg-cheese with your hands or the back of an oiled spoon and leave to cool completely.

The veg-cheese is now ready: cut into slices and serve with fresh vegetables.

Cream of Chickpea and Sesame

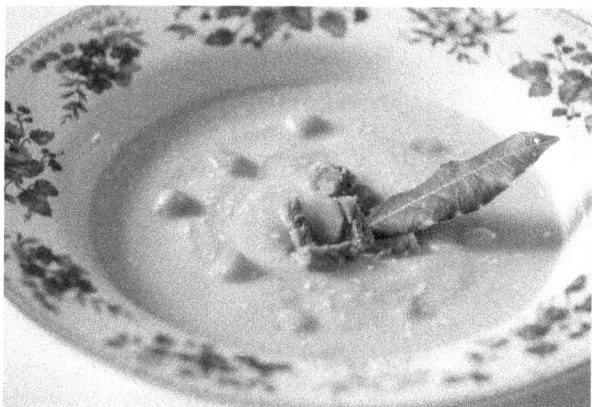

Recipe ID card

- 182 Kcal calories per serving
- Difficulty fairly easy
- Serves 10
- Preparation 105 minutes
- Average cost
- 15 minutes to prepare the sauce; 90 minutes to cook the chickpeas + 24 hours to soak them

Ingredients

For the hummus

- 150 g of chickpeas
- 1 sprig of parsley
- 1 clove of garlic
- salt to taste
- 1 pinch of chilli pepper
- about 30-50 ml of water
- 3 tablespoons (30 ml) of extra virgin olive oil
- untreated lemon juice
- 10 g (1 tablespoon) of tahina

To serve

- a few mint leaves
- 1 sprinkling of sweet paprika
- 2 pieces of pita or unleavened bread

Material Required

- Bowl for soaking chickpeas
- Casserole for cooking chickpeas
- Food processor
- Frying pan
- Wooden spoon
- Gravy boat or serving bowl

Preparation

Drain the chickpeas from the soaking water and rinse them in fresh running water to remove all the anti-nutritional elements.

Plunge the chickpeas into lightly salted boiling water and cook for about an hour and a half, until tender.

Drain the chickpeas from the water and flavour them in a pan with a little extra virgin olive oil, a clove of garlic and a little chilli pepper. If necessary, add more salt.

Remove the garlic clove from the chickpeas.

Transfer the seasoned chickpeas to a food processor, add the tahina, lemon juice and parsley.

If the hummus is too thick, add a little water from the chickpeas' cooking time: this will make the sauce more velvety and less compact.

Serve the hummus (the chickpea cream) with a sprinkling of sweet paprika, a few mint leaves and unleavened bread.

Savoury Water Muffins with Nettles

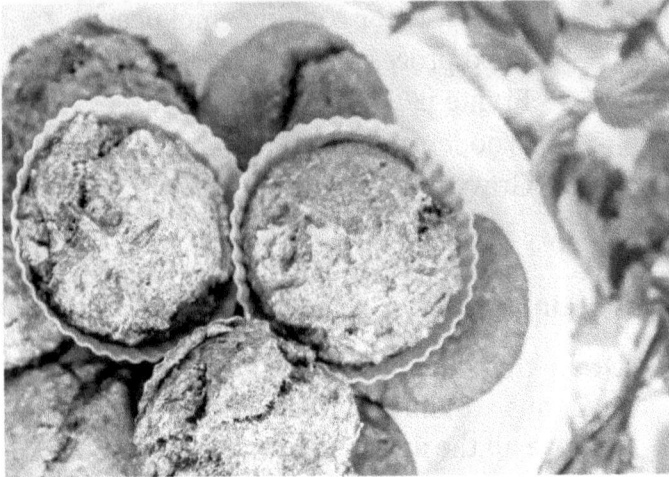

Recipe ID card

~ 150 Kcal calories per serving
~ Difficulty fairly easy
~ Serves 8
~ Preparation 25 minutes
~ Low cost
~ 15 minutes to prepare nettles; 10 minutes to prepare muffins; 25 minutes to bake

Ingredients

For 6 muffins

~ 200 g fresh spinach or nettles
~ 100 g wholemeal flour
~ 40 ml of corn seed oil
~ 150-170 ml water
~ 2 g of guar gum
~ 2 g of cream of tartar
~ 1 g of baking soda
~ 1 pinch of garlic powder
~ salt

Material Required

~ Basin for washing nettles
~ Muffin mold
~ Paper or silicone ramekins
~ Hand blender
~ Sieve
~ Food scale
~ Skimmer

Preparation

Cleaning Nettles. Wearing heavy-duty latex gloves, rinse nettles in cold water and immerse in a bowl filled with water and baking soda, which is essential for removing impurities. Rinse again.

Blanch nettles in plenty of boiling water for a couple of minutes.

Drain the nettles using a skimmer and collect them in a beaker. Add the cold water, a pinch of salt, the garlic powder, the oil and blend to a cream.

In a bowl, sift the whole wheat flour, add the guar gum, cream of tartar and baking soda (the basic ingredients of homemade chemical yeast) and, in the center, pour the mixture of water, oil and nettles.

Line a muffin mold with the ramekins provided.

Spread the mixture into the muffin cups, filling the cups up to 3/4 full.

Bake the muffins in a 160°C oven (ventilated mode) for 20-25 minutes or until golden brown.

Remove from oven and serve as desired. Those who wish can cut the muffins in half and stuff them as desired.

Goat Cheese and Strawberry Balls

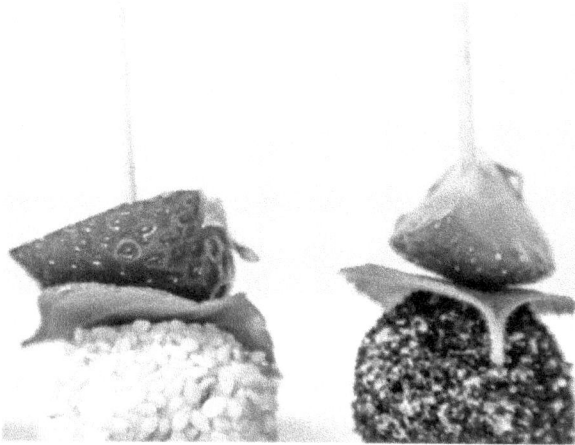

Recipe ID card

- ~ 204 Kcal calories per serving
- ~ Easy difficulty
- ~ Serves 4
- ~ Preparation 15 minutes
- ~ Low cost
- ~ 15 minutes + 1 hour cooling time

Ingredients

For the balls

- ~ 150 g of goat cheese
- ~ 100 g of strawberries
- ~ a few mint leaves
- ~ 1 pinch of pepper
- ~ 1 sprig of parsley
- ~ 1 pinch of salt

To serve

- ~ about 20 g of poppy seeds
- ~ about 20 g of sesame seeds
- ~ about 50 g of strawberries

Material Required

- ~ Food cutting board
- ~ Knife
- ~ Small bowls of various sizes
- ~ Toothpick
- ~ Wooden spoon
- ~ Spoons
- ~ Latex gloves

Preparation

Wash the strawberries well in cold water, then dry them with a soft cloth and remove the stems. Cut the strawberries into very small pieces.

Pour the goat cheese into a bowl and cream it with the chopped strawberries. Season with salt and pepper.

Chop up the parsley and mint, then add the herbs to the cream of goat cheese and strawberries. Let the cream rest in the refrigerator for at least 60 minutes: in this way, it will be easier to make small balls.

When it is cold and compact, take a small amount of cream with two teaspoons and make small balls, using your hands protected by latex gloves: the result will be about 20-25 balls.

Roll one half of the balls in sesame seeds and the remaining in poppy seeds.

Cut the strawberries (for decoration) into quarters. Stick each ball into a toothpick and finish with a quarter of a strawberry and a mint leaf.

Serve the balls well chilled.

Broad Beans Pesto

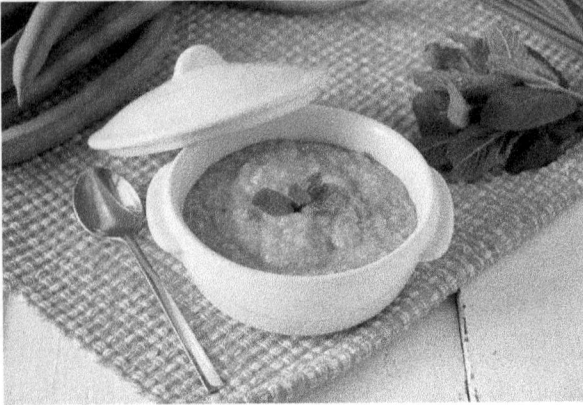

Peel a clove of garlic, cut it in half and remove the undigestible center.

Cut the pecorino cheese into cubes and combine in the blender with the broad beans, pine nuts (optional) and garlic. Flavor with mint leaves and a pinch of salt: blend intermittently adding as much oil as necessary until you get the consistency of a cream. To avoid adding too much oil, it is advisable to mix the cream with one or two tablespoons of cold water.

Fava bean pesto is ready and can be immediately used to season pasta, to prepare excellent bruschetta or to accompany pinzimonio, meat and fish.

If it is not to be consumed immediately, it is advisable to keep the fava bean sauce in the fridge for 3-4 days, taking care to cover the surface with a little oil; alternatively, keep it in the freezer for a couple of months.

Recipe ID card

- ~ 235 Kcal calories per serving
- ~ Easy difficulty
- ~ Serves 4
- ~ Preparation 15 minutes
- ~ Low cost

Ingredients

- ~ Raw, shelled, fresh food: 200 g of broad beans
- ~ 50 g of pecorino cheese
- ~ 1 garlic clove
- ~ A few mint leaves
- ~ 4-5 tablespoons of extra virgin olive oil
- ~ salt
- ~ Optional: 10 g of pine nuts

Material Required

- ~ Blender or mortar
- ~ Bowl
- ~ Spoon

Preparation

Shell fresh fava beans from the pod and peel them to remove the hard, woody integument.

Sauce Tzatziki

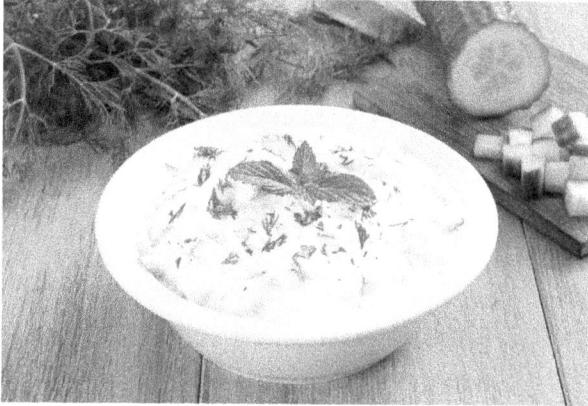

Recipe ID card

- ~ 53 Kcal calories per serving
- ~ Easy difficulty
- ~ Serves 6
- ~ Preparation 10 minutes
- ~ Average cost
- ~ 10 minutes + 1 hour for draining

Ingredients

For the sauce

- ~ 340 g of Greek yogurt
- ~ a few mint leaves
- ~ 1 teaspoon of oregano
- ~ 1 tablespoon of extra virgin olive oil
- ~ Optional: 1 pinch of pepper
- ~ 1 pinch of salt
- ~ 1 clove of garlic
- ~ 1 teaspoon untreated lemon juice
- ~ 200 g (1 medium) of cucumbers

To serve

- ~ 1 handful of black olives
- ~ A few slices of cucumber

Material Required

- ~ Manual or electric grater
- ~ Colander
- ~ Bowls
- ~ Wooden spoon
- ~ Mortar and pestle (or spoon)
- ~ Vegetable peeler

Preparation

Wash a cucumber and peel it with the help of a vegetable peeler, then grate the pulp with an electric or manual grater.

Put the grated pulp of the cucumber in a colander and let it drain for at least 40-50 minutes. At the end, you will get a very dry product.

Crush a clove of garlic in a mortar together with some mint leaves until obtaining a cream. However, it is not recommended to mince the garlic and mint in a blender.

Pour the Greek yoghurt into a bowl, add salt, pepper (optional), lemon juice and a tablespoon of extra virgin olive oil.

Flavor the sauce with oregano to taste.

Serve the tzatziki sauce decorating with black olives and cucumber slices, perhaps accompanying with pita bread.

Tuna Tartare

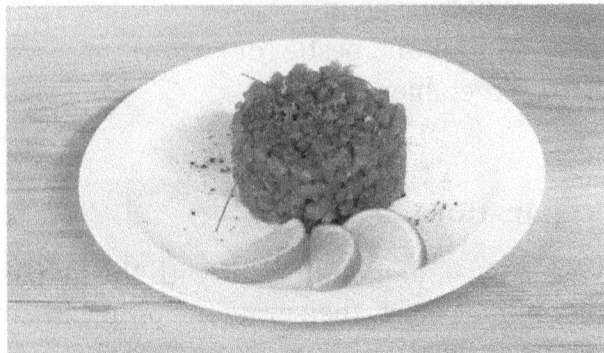

Recipe ID card

- ~ 217 Kcal calories per serving
- ~ Easy difficulty
- ~ Serves 2
- ~ Preparation 15 minutes
- ~ Average cost

Ingredients for 2 people

- ~ 200 g of fresh tuna
- ~ 1 piece of ginger
- ~ 2 tablespoons of extra virgin olive oil
- ~ 1 pinch of pepper
- ~ 1 pinch of salt
- ~ dill or fennel
- ~ 5 g of flax seeds
- ~ 5 g of sesame seeds
- ~ 20 g (about 3) squash blossoms

For decoration (optional)

- ~ A few stalks of chives

Material Required

- ~ Pasta cup with a diameter of 10 cm
- ~ Cutting board
- ~ Knife
- ~ Bowls
- ~ Grater

Preparation

Cut the raw tuna into small cubes, avoiding over-stressing the fibres of the meat.

Clean the squash blossoms, then remove the pistil and the lower end. Cut the zucchini flowers into thin strips.

Pour the tuna tartare into a bowl and add the squash blossom strips, flax seeds and sesame seeds. Flavor with fresh peeled and grated ginger, chopped fresh fennel (or dill), oil, salt and pepper.

Pour the mixture into a pastry cup (cookie cutter) to give the tartare a round or square shape. Serve decorating with a few stems of chives.

Savoury Pie with Ricotta and Tuna

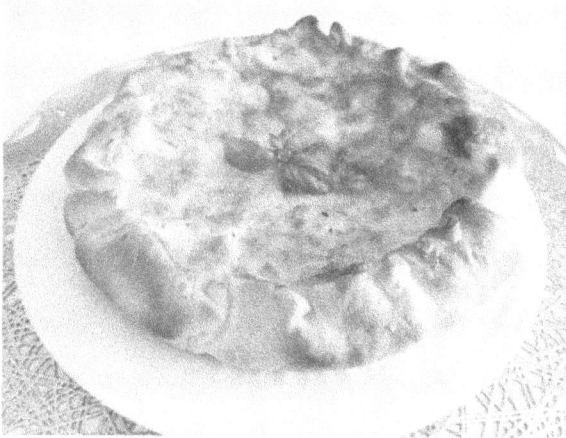

Recipe ID card

~ 188 Kcal calories per serving
~ Easy difficulty
~ Serves 6
~ Preparation 40 minutes
~ Low cost
~ 10 minutes for preparation + 25-30 minutes for cooking

Ingredients

For the dough

~ 160 g of drained tuna in oil
~ 30 g of black or green olives
~ 1 sprig of parsley
~ 5-6 fillets of anchovies or anchovies
~ 30 g of capers
~ 30 g of breadcrumbs
~ 30 g of grated Parmesan cheese
~ 120 g (2 medium-sized) eggs
~ 250 g of fresh ricotta

For the mold

~ 10 g butter (for the pan)
~ 10 g of breadcrumbs

Material Required

~ Bowls of various sizes
~ Wooden spoon
~ Star mold
~ Knives
~ Brush

Preparation

In a large bowl, pour the tuna, breadcrumbs and ricotta cheese: mix well.

Add the eggs, one at a time, and continue to mix the ingredients.

In the meantime, chop the parsley rather coarsely, and add it to the ricotta mixture.

Then proceed by adding the olives, anchovies in pieces and desalted capers.

Amalgamate the mixture well. Finally, add the grated grana cheese. It is not necessary to add salt because the ingredients are already tasty.

In the meantime, preheat the oven and butter a star-shaped mold with a little melted butter. Sprinkle the mold with a little breadcrumbs, which is essential to help the mixture come away from the pan.

Pour the mixture into the mould, level with a spoon and bake for 25-30 minutes at 180°C.

Turn the mold out onto a serving plate, decorate as desired and serve hot.

Vegetables and Salads for Diabetics

Artichokes Trifoliated

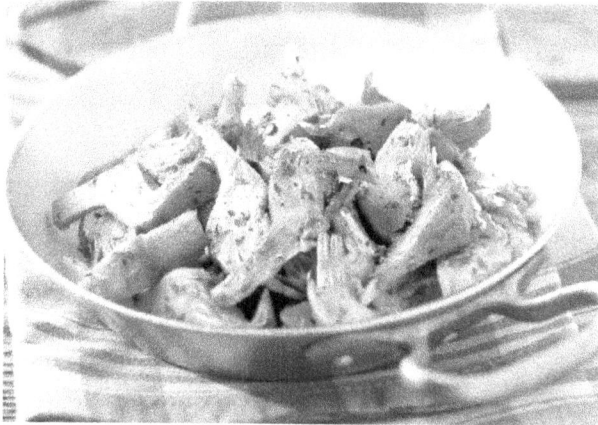

Recipe ID card

- ~ 70 Kcal calories per serving
- ~ Difficulty quite easy
- ~ Serves 4
- ~ Preparation 45 minutes
- ~ Average cost
- ~ 15 minutes for cleaning + 30 minutes for cooking

Ingredients

- ~ 1 bunch of 800 g (5 pieces) of artichokes
- ~ 50 ml of dry white wine
- ~ Optional: 1 teaspoon (5 g) rice flour
- ~ Optional: Grated zest of untreated lemon
- ~ 1 tuft of parsley
- ~ 1 clove of garlic
- ~ pepper
- ~ salt
- ~ 2 tablespoons of extra virgin olive oil
- ~ about 100 ml of water

Material Required

- ~ Bowl with water and lemon
- ~ Latex gloves (optional)
- ~ Ceramic knives
- ~ Saucepan with lid
- ~ Wooden spoon

Preparation

Carefully clean the artichokes

Heat a couple of tablespoons of e.v.o. oil in a casserole, adding the garlic, either minced or poached.

Pour the artichoke slices - well drained from the soaking water - into the hot oil.

Season with salt and pepper to taste. Deglaze with the dry white wine and, once the alcohol has evaporated, add a little water. Wait for the boiling and cook for about 20-30 minutes, or until the artichokes are soft.

When cooked, raise the heat to brown them slightly. Dissolve the rice starch in one or two tablespoons of water, then pour the thickener directly into the saucepan: in this way, you will obtain a thick and creamy artichoke sauce.

Finish with a generous handful of chopped parsley, continue cooking for another 2-3 minutes and serve, adding the grated rind of an organic lemon to taste.

Cauliflower In Oil

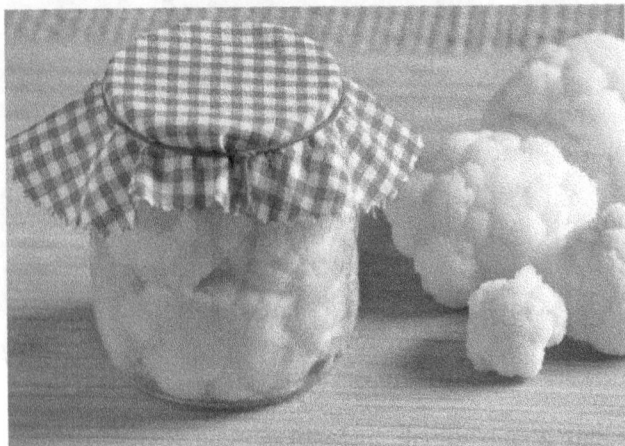

Recipe ID card

~ 112 Kcal calories per serving
~ Difficulty fairly easy
~ Serves 15 people
~ Preparation 60 minutes
~ Average cost
~ 60 minutes + 8 hours for drying

Ingredients

~ 1 kg of cleaned cauliflower florets
~ 1 litre of vinegar
~ 1 liter of dry white wine
~ salt
~ 1 tablespoon of peppercorns
~ 1 tablespoon of coriander grains
~ 1 tablespoon of mustard seeds

Material Required

~ Pasta drainer
~ Glass jars with screw caps
~ Large saucepan
~ Skimmer
~ Clean dishcloth
~ Knife
~ Cutting board
~ Bowls
~ Food thermometer

Preparation

First of all, carefully wash all the utensils needed to make the preserve: jars, pots, colander, chopping board, knife etc..

Clean the cauliflower: remove the ribs and leaves, then remove the inflorescences and cut them into pieces about the same size.

Wash the inflorescences in water and bicarbonate of soda, rubbing them gently to remove any trace of soil and impurities. Rinse cauliflower again in cold water.

Prepare a solution composed of decolorized wine vinegar and white wine in equal parts. Bring to a boil, add a pinch of salt and dip the cauliflower florets in it. Cook the cauliflower for 3 minutes, beginning at the boil.

Drain the cauliflower on a colander, then transfer the tops to a clean dish towel and leave to dry overnight.

The next day, prepare the glass jars with their screw caps. Place the jars in a large saucepan and fill with water. Put on fire and calculate at least 20 minutes from boiling.

Remove jars from boiling water and let them dry for few minutes: they must not contain any trace of water. Pour a little oil into the jars, flavor with dry spices as desired (e.g. coriander seeds, mustard seeds, peppercorns or chili pepper, parsley, basil, garlic, thyme, oregano, etc.) and fill with cauliflower, alternating with oil and flavourings. Proceed in this manner until the jar is completely filled.

Using a spatula, gently crush the cauliflowers covered with oil in order to release the air bubbles that inevitably formed when the jar was filled with oil. Wait a few hours and check the oil level: if it has dropped below that of the vegetables, proceed with topping up (further addition of oil).

Close the jars with their respective caps and proceed with pasteurization at 80°C for 10 minutes. Then place the jars in a saucepan, taking care to place a tea towel to avoid chipping the jars during pasteurization. Allow 10 minutes from the time the jars reach 80°C (176°F), monitoring the temperature frequently with a thermometer.

Allow the canning jars to cool in the water until a vacuum is reached.

Store jars in the dark for 6 months to 1 year. In order to appreciate the flavor at its best, it is recommended to consume the preserve at least 1 month after potting.

Grana Cheese Baskets Stuffed with Bulgur Salad

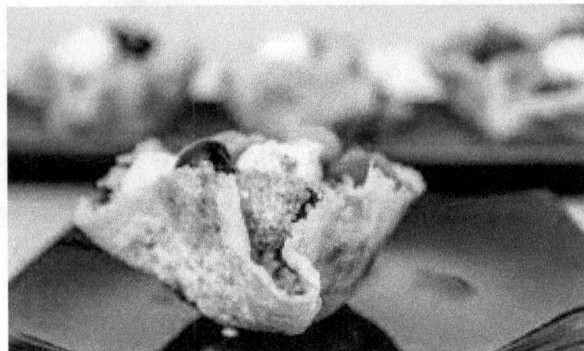

Recipe ID card

- ~ 194 Kcal calories per serving
- ~ Difficulty fairly easy
- ~ Serves 4
- ~ Preparation 30 minutes
- ~ Average cost
- ~ 10 minutes for baskets; 10 minutes to cook bulgur; 10 minutes to prepare salad

Ingredients

For 4 baskets

- ~ About 100 g of grated Parmesan cheese

For the accompanying sauce

- ~ 70 g of tomatoes or coppery tomatoes
- ~ 15 g of pine nuts
- ~ Salt and pepper to taste
- ~ 2 tablespoons of extra virgin olive oil
- ~ 20 g of capers
- ~ 2 tablespoons of water
- ~ 30 g of rocket

For the bulgur salad

- ~ 1 tablespoon of extra virgin olive oil
- ~ 50 g of mozzarella cherries
- ~ 50 g of green olives
- ~ 50 g of black olives
- ~ 50 g of cherry tomatoes

- ~ 200 ml of water
- ~ 100 g of bulgur

Material Required

- ~ Small bowls or narrow-bottomed glasses
- ~ Stone or non-stick frying pan
- ~ Immersion mixer
- ~ High-sided container (beaker)
- ~ Baking paper
- ~ Saucepan for cooking bulgur
- ~ Chopping board
- ~ Knives
- ~ Bowls
- ~ Scoop

Preparation

First, cook the bulgur in lightly salted water: for optimal cooking, pour the bulgur into the boiling water, then turn off the heat and cover with the lid until the water is completely absorbed. 10 minutes will be enough.

In the meantime prepare the grana baskets, which will be the "cups" on which we will then serve the bulgur. Heat a stone or non-stick pan on the stove: place a rectangle of parchment paper on top, then pour a handful of grated Parmesan cheese (about 25-30 g), trying to form an even and rather thin layer. After a few moments, a golden crust will form. At this point, place another sheet of parchment paper on top and gently turn the mixture over so that the crust forms on the other side as well.

After a few moments, the parmesan disk will begin to brown on the other side as well: quickly remove from the heat (with the baking paper) and pour the slightly solidified parmesan over the bottom of a narrow glass or a cold bowl. Leave to cool for a few moments: the change in temperature will help the cheese to solidify and take on the shape of the container.

Prepare the accompanying sauce for the bulgur. In an immersion blender pour the arugula, chopped tomato, pine nuts, oil, salt, pepper, water and capers: blend well to obtain a velvety sauce.

After about ten minutes, the bulgur will have absorbed all the water: therefore crumble the mixture with the help of a wooden spoon. Pour the bulgur into a bowl with a drop of oil to prevent the bulgur grains from sticking together.

Season the bulgur with the chopped cherry tomatoes, black olives and green olives. Add the mozzarellas only when the bulgur has cooled completely to avoid melting the cheese.

Distribute the bulgur salad in the baskets with a few drops of sauce and serve.

How to Clean and Cook Celeriac

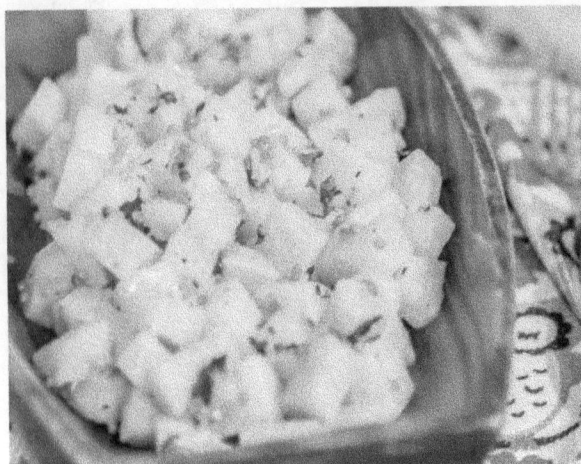

Recipe ID card

~ Easy difficulty
~ Serves 4
~ Preparation 10 minutes
~ Low cost
~ 10 minutes for preparation; 15 minutes for cooking

Ingredients

~ 500 g of celeriac
~ 2 spoons of extra virgin olive oil
~ salt
~ pepper
~ parsley
~ Optional: 1 tablespoon of mustard seeds

Material Required

~ Brush
~ Cutting board
~ Knife
~ Frying pan
~ Scoop or wooden spoon

Preparation

Wash the root thoroughly, taking care to rub the surface with a brush in order to remove impurities and traces of soil. Cut celeriac root in half or in quarters, then remove peel with a knife.

Cut the root into slices a couple of centimetres thick. From each slice, cut strips and then dices of regular size.

Heat a frying pan and add a couple of tablespoons of extra virgin olive oil. Add the diced celeriac, season with salt and pepper and, if desired, add a tablespoon of mustard seeds.

Keep a lively flame for 2-3 minutes, then lower the flame, cover with the lid and continue cooking for 10-15 minutes, until the celeriac will be soft but firm.

Turn off the flame and flavor with parsley.

How to Clean Artichokes

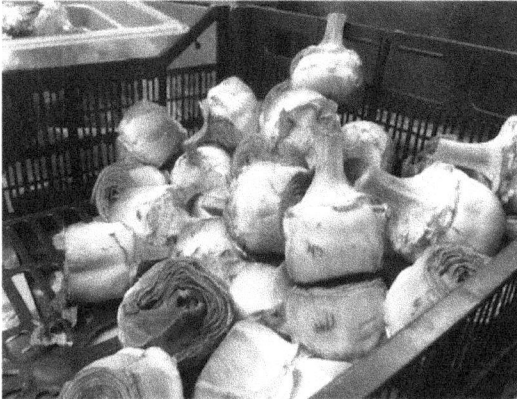

Recipe ID card

~ 28 Kcal calories per serving
~ Difficulty fairly easy
~ Serves 4
~ Preparation 15 minutes
~ Average cost

Ingredients

~ About 750 g (5 large) artichokes
~ Untreated lemon juice
~ Water

Material Required

~ Bowl
~ Knives preferably ceramic
~ Latex gloves (optional)
~ Vegetable peeler
~ Digger

Preparation

First of all prepare a solution of cold water and lemon juice: artichokes tend to oxidize very quickly and the citric acid contained in lemon slows down the process.

It is advisable to wear latex gloves or to rub half a lemon on the skin of hands in order to prevent them from turning black.

Begin by cleaning the artichokes. Cut the stem (caul) of the artichoke about 4 inches from the receptacle (heart) or where it is soft.

Peel the stem with a ceramic knife or vegetable peeler to remove the tougher, woody outer filaments. Cut the stem into rounds and dip them in acidulated water.

Remove the outer leaves (bracts) with your hands until they are soft to the touch. Remove the top part of the artichoke (3-4 cm from the tip) with a knife.

Cut the artichoke in half (lengthwise): in the center you can see the typical inedible beard (called "hay" or "pappo"): remove it with a sharp knife or a small digger.

Cut the artichoke into thin slices, then dip them in acidulated water. After that, you can proceed with cooking: artichokes can be boiled, steamed, baked or cooked in a pan. Check out the recipe for artichoke sauce.

To get artichoke bottoms instead, you will have to proceed in another way. After removing the stem, cut off the ends of the bracts (3-4 cm). Open the artichoke with your hands until you reach the center. Remove the beard with the help of a small digger, then immediately plunge the artichoke into acidulated water.

Cleaning Mushrooms

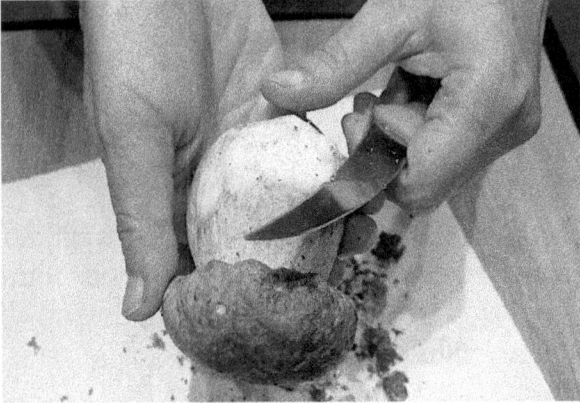

Recipe ID card

~ 21 Kcal calories per serving
~ Easy difficulty
~ Serves 4
~ Preparation 30 minutes
~ Average cost

Ingredients

~ about 750 g of chanterelles, porcini or champignon mushrooms or chiodini or pioppini

Material Required

~ Cutting board
~ Knife preferably ceramic
~ Damp dishcloth or paper towel

Preparation

Cleaning Champignon Mushrooms

First cut off the end of the stem to remove traces of soil. Gently peel off the stem by performing a twisting motion. Remove the skin covering the chapel, starting from the edges towards the center. Cut the cap into thin slices and the stem into rounds or thin slices.

Cleaning Porcini Mushrooms

With a sharp knife, remove traces of soil and impurities starting from the end of the stem, taking care to remove as little pulp as possible. Scrape the surface with the knife to facilitate the operation. Repeat the scraping also in the part of the chapel. It is not recommended to wash the mushroom in water because, as it behaves like a sponge, it tends to fill up with water. Anyway, in case the mushroom is very difficult to clean and the soil remains even after having dabbed it with a damp cloth, it is suggested to pass it quickly in cold running water.

If the porcini mushroom is small, cut it whole in slices (lengthwise). If the size of the mushroom is important, it is advisable to detach the cap from the stalk by making a delicate rotating movement and to obtain thin gills from the head and the stalk.

Cleaning Chanterelle Mushrooms

Cleaning chanterelle mushrooms is not difficult but it is important to remove every trace of soil, which tends to get stuck between the gills of the mushroom (inner part of the chapel). With the tip of a knife, patiently remove the impurities hiding between the gills of the mushroom; scrape (if necessary) the surface of the stem and remove the end. Using a damp cloth, gently rub the top of the head. If the mushroom is large, cut it into segments lengthwise; if it is small, it can be cooked whole (without cutting it into pieces).

Mushrooms Trifoliated

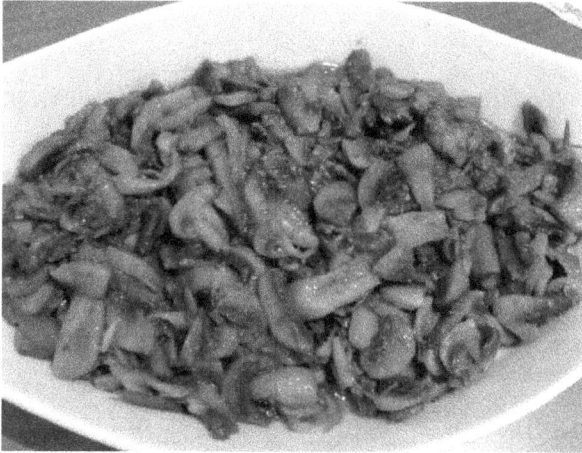

Recipe ID card

~ 43 Kcal calories per serving
~ Easy difficulty
~ Serves 4
~ Preparation 20 minutes
~ Average cost
~ 20 minutes + time for cleaning mushrooms

Ingredients

~ 750 g of champignon or chiodini or pioppini mushrooms
~ Plenty of parsley
~ salt
~ pepper
~ 2 tablespoons (20 ml) of extra virgin olive oil
~ 1 clove of garlic

Material Required

~ Cutting board
~ Knife preferably ceramic
~ Saucepan with lid
~ Wooden spoon or spatula
~ Garlic toothpick (optional)

Preparation

Clean the mushrooms (in this case we chose porcini, chanterelles and champignons) taking care to remove all traces of soil and impurities. Cut the mushrooms into fairly even slices for even cooking.

Heat 2 tablespoons of extra virgin olive oil and flavor with a clove of poached garlic: it is advisable to pierce the garlic with a toothpick to facilitate its subsequent removal.

Now proceed with cooking the mushrooms: brown the chanterelle mushrooms in the oil over very high heat and without a lid, taking care to stir often to avoid burning them. Continue cooking for 10 minutes.

After this time, add the other mushrooms and cook over moderate heat for another 10 minutes.

At this point, season with salt and pepper. Chop some parsley and add it to the mushrooms. Stir and allow the cooking liquid to dry up (only if necessary).

Remove the garlic clove and serve.

Alpha Alpha Sprouts

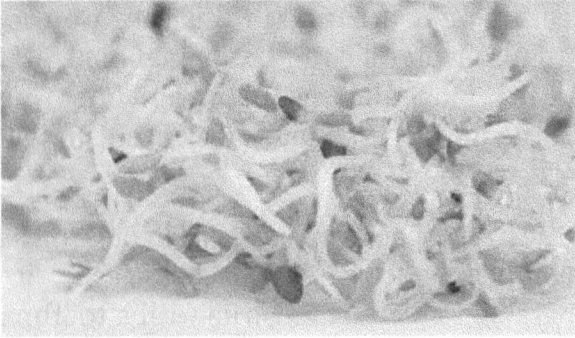

Recipe ID card

~ 60 Kcal calories per serving
~ Difficulty fairly easy
~ Serves 4
~ Preparation 10 minutes
~ Low cost
~ 10 minutes to prepare; 6 hours to soak; 5-6 days to germinate

Ingredients

~ 1 tablespoon (about 20 g) alpha seeds
~ water

Material Required

~ Glass jars
~ Strainer
~ Bowls
~ Gauze
~ Elastic or food string

Preparation

First of all, soak alpha seeds in cold water for 4-6 hours. After the soaking time, it can be noticed seeds appear swollen and the skin enclosing them (tegument) begins to split: seeds are ready to sprout.

Drain seeds from soaking and put them in a large glass jar. Rinse a couple of times, removing the water.

Cover the glass jar with gauze, then seal with a rubber band or kitchen string.

Set the jar upside down, placing the jar gauze side down on a colander. Place the strainer over a bowl, so that water droplets collect in the container below.

Repeat twice a day.

After 3 days from soaking, it is advisable to expose the jar with the partially sprouted seeds to the sun: light, in fact, activates chlorophyll and enriches the young seedlings.

After 4-5 days, it is possible to notice evident sprouts, ready to be eaten.

Alpha alpha sprouts can be consumed raw, steamed or sautéed in a pan. However, in order to fully benefit from their properties, it is recommended to eat them raw. Alfalfa sprouts are in fact rich in vitamins C, D, E, K, vitamins of group B and minerals such as zinc, selenium, magnesium, calcium and phosphor. They are rich in coumestrol (phytoestrogenic properties) and chlorophyll (antioxidant properties). They have a delicate flavor that goes well with countless foods.

Sprouts can be stored in the refrigerator for 5-7 days.

Cedar and Sprouts Salad

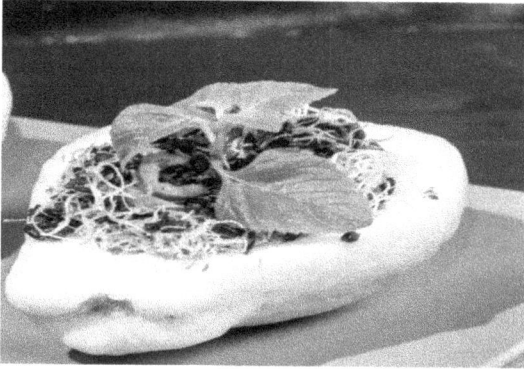

Recipe ID card

~ 114 Kcal calories per serving
~ Difficulty fairly easy
~ Serves 2
~ Preparation 20 minutes
~ Average cost
~ 20 minutes for preparation; 40 minutes for cooking rice

Ingredients

~ 500 g of citrons
~ 50 g of alpha shoots
~ 50 g of Venus rice
~ A few mint leaves
~ 2 tablespoons of extra virgin olive oil
~ 30 g of green olives
~ 20 g of sunflower seeds
~ salt

Material Required

~ Digger
~ Saucepan for cooking rice
~ Cutting board
~ Bowl

Preparation

First, prepare the alpha alpha sprouts.

Dedicate yourself to cooking the Venere rice. Plunge the rice into lightly salted boiling water and cook over very low heat for about 40 minutes, following the cooking directions on the package.

Drain the Venere rice from the cooking water and allow to cool.

Meanwhile, coarsely chop the mint and cut the olives into rounds.

Cut the citron in half and squeeze out the juice. Remove part of the zest, chop and set aside.

Hollow out the pulp of the citron: it will serve as a container for the salad.

Dress the rice with oil, olives, sunflower seeds, sprouts, chopped mint, juice and zest of the citron.

Fill the cedar bowl with the salad and serve immediately.

Light Chicken Salad

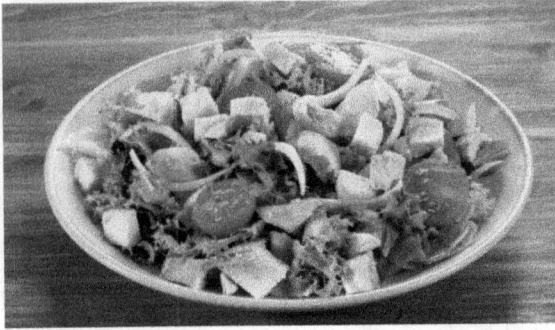

Recipe ID card

- ~ 93 Kcal calories per serving
- ~ Difficulty very easy
- ~ Serves 4
- ~ Preparation 20 minutes
- ~ Low cost

Ingredients

For the chicken salad

- ~ pepper
- ~ 10 g of gomasio
- ~ 2 tablespoons of extra virgin olive oil
- ~ Lime juice
- ~ 50 g of corn
- ~ 200 g of tender salad
- ~ 200 g of grapes
- ~ 350 g of chicken breast

For the accompanying sauce

- ~ a few stalks of chives
- ~ 1 teaspoon of mustard
- ~ 125 g low-fat yoghurt

Material Required

- ~ Frying pan
- ~ Bowl
- ~ Cutting board
- ~ Knife

Preparation

Prepare the grilled chicken. Heat a frying pan very hot and, without adding oil or other seasonings, sear the chicken on both sides. Once a golden crust has formed, cover the pan with the lid, lower the heat and cook for 5-6 minutes.

Remove the steak from the pan and return to a cutting board. Cut the chicken breast into thin strips.

Until the chicken cools, clean the grapes, wash the berries and dry them. Cut the grapes in half and remove the inner seeds.

Wash the salad and drain it of excess water.

Prepare the accompanying yogurt sauce. In a bowl, mix the low-fat natural yogurt with the mustard sauce and chopped chives. Set aside.

In a bowl, combine the lettuce, corn and grapes. Prepare a citronette sauce by emulsifying the oil with the juice of one lime and the pepper.

Add the cold chicken strips to the salad and season with gomasio.

Summer Protein Salad with Snails

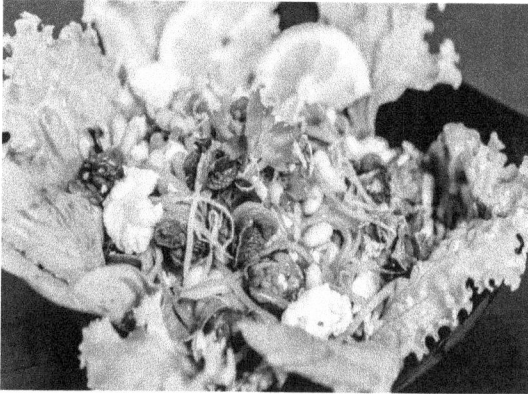

Recipe ID card

- ~ 154 Kcal calories per serving
- ~ Easy difficulty
- ~ Serves 4
- ~ Preparation 30 minutes
- ~ Average cost
- ~ 30 minutes for preparation + 3 hours for cooking the snails + 8 hours for soaking the soybeans

Ingredients

For the salad

- ~ Frozen, cleaned and shelled product: 400 g of snails
- ~ 30 g of almonds
- ~ 120 g of egg white
- ~ 100 g of dried yellow soybeans
- ~ 150 g of carrots

For the seasoning

- ~ salt
- ~ 1 tablespoon of pink peppercorns
- ~ A few stalks of chives
- ~ 2 tablespoons of extra virgin olive oil
- ~ Juice and zest of untreated lemon
- ~ 1 sprig of parsley

Material Required

- ~ Casseroles of various sizes
- ~ Bowls
- ~ Skimmer
- ~ Spoons
- ~ Frying pan
- ~ Scoop
- ~ Cutting board
- ~ Ceramic knife
- ~ Lemon line or grater

Preparation

First, soak the yellow soybeans overnight. Rinse them in cold water to remove any anti-nutritional elements and boil them in water for an hour or more, until soft. Drain the soybeans and set aside.

Meanwhile, thaw the snails and rinse them in cold water.

Boil the snails in plenty of lightly salted water. We recommend cooking for about 3 hours: the longer they cook, the softer the snail meat will be.

Remove the snails from the cooking water, using a skimmer.

Peel the carrot and grate it finely.

Prepare the "omelette" of egg whites. Beat the egg whites quickly with a fork, adding a pinch of salt. Grease a frying pan with a little oil and scramble the egg whites, turning them often with a paddle.

Toast the almonds in a frying pan, taking care not to burn them.

Prepare the salad dressing. Finely chop a few stems of chives and chop the parsley. Grate the zest of an organic lemon and set aside. In a bowl, prepare a sort of citronette sauce by emulsifying the oil with plenty of lemon juice. Adjust the salt, add the chopped chives, plenty of parsley, pink peppercorns and grated lemon zest.

Mix the cooked snails with the soybeans, scrambled egg whites, grated carrots and season with the freshly prepared emulsion.

Arrange the escargot and soybean salad on a serving plate and finish with the toasted almonds.

Low Fat Lentils

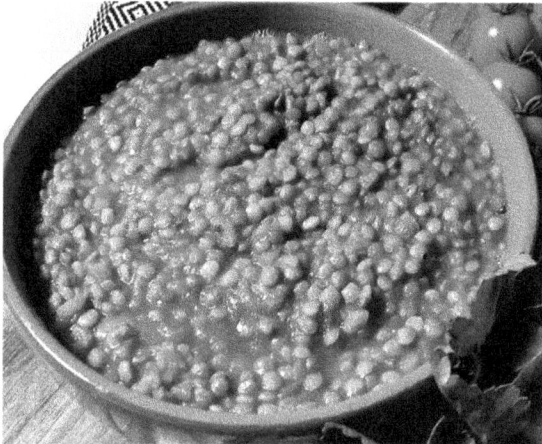

Recipe ID card

~ 133 Kcal calories per serving
~ Easy difficulty
~ Serves 6
~ Preparation 90 minutes
~ Low cost
~ 90 minutes + soaking time

Ingredients

~ 250 g of dried lentils
~ 1 pinch of salt
~ 1 pinch of pepper
~ 2 tablespoons of extra virgin olive oil
~ 1 clove of garlic
~ 1 teaspoon of tomato paste
~ About 100 g of carrots
~ 300 ml vegetable stock
~ Optional: 1 bay leaf
~ 1 celery rib

Material Required

~ Bowl
~ Saucepan with lid
~ Electric blender
~ Vegetable peeler
~ Pasta strainer or colander
~ Wooden spoon

Preparation

First, soak the lentils. Pour the dried legumes into a large bowl and cover with plenty of cold water. Leave the lentils to soak for at least 10-12 hours, until they have tripled their volume.

At this point, rinse the lentils in cold water to remove all the anti-nutritional elements contained in the seeds.

Clean the vegetables: wash and peel the carrots and cut them into small pieces. Wash the celery and cut it into small pieces. Chop the vegetables in a mixer.

Brown the chopped vegetables in a saucepan, adding 2 tablespoons of oil, a tablespoon of tomato paste and a clove of garlic.

Pour the rinsed lentils into a saucepan and cover the surface with the hot vegetable stock. Cook for 1 1/2 to 2 hours, depending on the type of lentils chosen. It is recommended to check the lentils often during cooking: if the liquid evaporates too much, add a few more ladles of broth.

When the lentils are soft, add salt and pepper to taste and season with a bay leaf. Continue cooking for another 5 minutes.

Not fried eggplants Parmigiana style

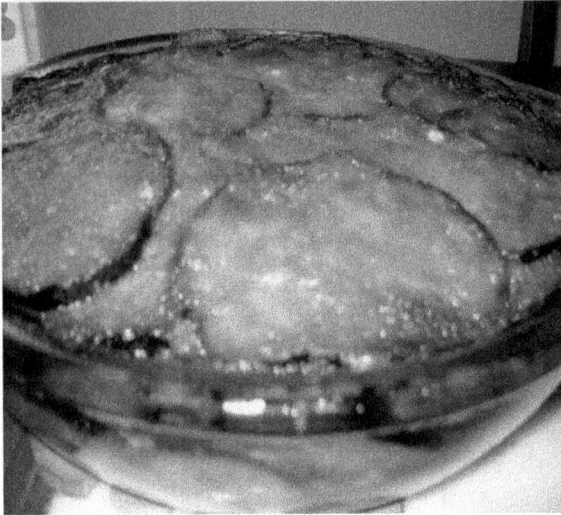

Recipe ID card

~ 78 Kcal calories per serving
~ Difficulty fairly easy
~ Serves 5
~ Preparation 50 minutes
~ Low cost
~ 15 minutes to cook eggplant; 10 minutes to prepare parmigiana; 20-25 minutes to bake

Ingredients

~ For 9-10 mini pies
~ 600 g (2 large) eggplants
~ 170 g of provola or mozzarella cheese
~ 300 g (2 large) coppery tomatoes
~ 80 g of tomato puree
~ 10-15 basil leaves
~ about 30 g of grated Parmesan cheese
~ about 2 tablespoons of extra virgin olive oil
~ salt
~ pepper

Material Required

~ Cutting board
~ Knives preferably ceramic
~ Cheese cutter knife
~ Large stone or non-stick frying pan
~ Small bowl
~ Brush
~ Pyrex dish
~ Cheese grater

Preparation

Wash the eggplant thoroughly, removing the inedible end. With a knife (preferably ceramic), cut into rounds about 1 cm thick.

Put a very large, shallow pan on the stove: when it is very hot, blanch the eggplant slices without adding seasoning. For optimal cooking, it is advisable to cook them for about 2 minutes on each side over a high flame, avoiding browning them excessively: then lower the flame, cover with the lid and continue cooking for another 5 minutes, so that the heart can become soft.

Once ready, arrange the eggplants in a dish, pour a drizzle of oil and salt to taste.

Cut the cheese into thin slices. In the Neapolitan version, eggplants parmigiana (besides being fried) are prepared with mozzarella cheese. However, it is possible to replace mozzarella with provola cheese or with another cheese of your choice.

Cut also tomatoes in very thin slices, then salt and add some pepper to taste.

Season the tomato puree with salt, add a little chopped basil and a tablespoon of extra virgin olive oil. Distribute almost all the tomato puree on the bottom of a Pyrex dish.

Start preparing the eggplant pyramids. On a cutting board, place a slice of eggplant, cover with a slice of tomato, a slice of mozzarella, some basil and some grated Parmesan cheese; continue with another slice of eggplant, tomato, cheese, basil and cover with another eggplant.

Arrange the "pyramid" of eggplant on the baking dish. Proceed in this manner until the baking dish is filled.

At this point, arrange on all the eggplants a slice of mozzarella, a grating of grana cheese and cover with a teaspoon of tomato puree.

Bake the baking dish at 200°C for 20-30 minutes. Alternatively, you can also cook the parmigiana in the microwave, with the combined micro-grill function, for 5 minutes.

Serve the single portions with a small leaf of basil.

Pasta Salad

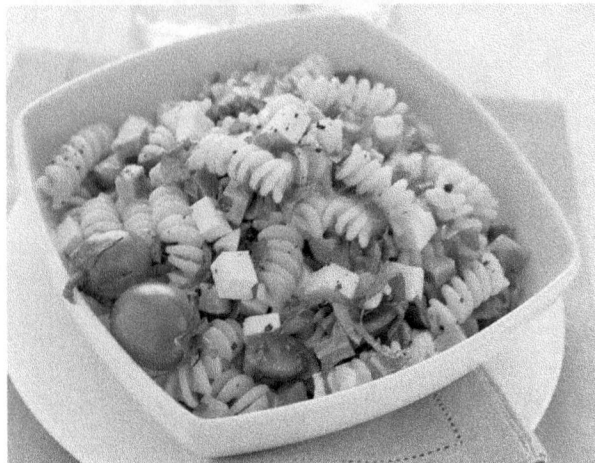

Recipe ID card

- ~ 176 Kcal calories per serving
- ~ Easy difficulty
- ~ Serves 4
- ~ Preparation 20 minutes
- ~ Low cost
- ~ 20 minutes to prepare; 1 hour to chill

Ingredients

- ~ 280 g of whole wheat pasta
- ~ pepper
- ~ salt
- ~ 100 g of Genovese pesto
- ~ 50 g of corn
- ~ 150 g of cherry tomatoes
- ~ 30 g of almonds
- ~ 30 g of sunflower seeds
- ~ Ready-to-eat, boiled food: 100 g of chickpeas
- ~ 100 g of mozzarella
- ~ 50 g of celery
- ~ A few leaves of parsley
- ~ 150 g of melon pulp
- ~ 1 teaspoon of oregano

Material Required

- ~ Casserole
- ~ Bowl
- ~ Cutting board
- ~ Knife
- ~ Pasta strainer
- ~ Digger

Preparation

Cook whole-wheat pasta in plenty of salted water, respecting the cooking time recommended on the package.

Meanwhile, prepare the dressing. In a pan, toast the chopped almonds and sunflower seeds to bring out their aroma, taking care to stir often and maintain a medium-sweet flame.

Wash the cherry tomatoes and dice them. Wash the celery, remove the hard filaments and cut it into strips.

Clean the melon, wash it in cold water to remove any traces of soil and remove the seeds using a spoon. With a small digger, obtain many small balls of melon and put aside. Alternatively, it is possible to cut the melon into cubes with a knife, after having removed the rind.

When the pasta is ready, drain it from the cooking water and pass it quickly under a jet of cold water: in this way, the cooking is stopped and the pasta will remain "al dente". Leave to cool.

Put the whole-wheat pasta in a bowl and flavor with homemade Genovese pesto and add pepper, celery, cherry tomatoes, chopped parsley, oregano, corn, boiled chickpeas, diced mozzarella and toasted almonds and sunflower seeds. Finish with the melon balls. Adjust salt if necessary.

Vegan Lentil Meatloaf

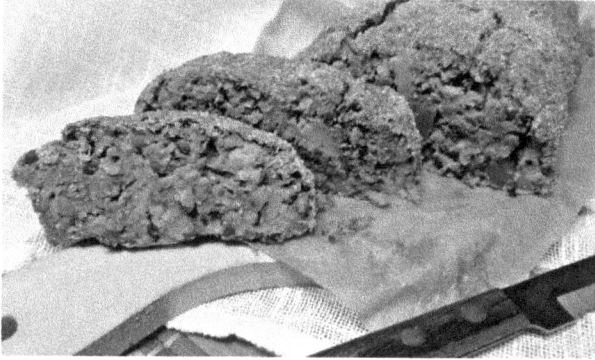

Recipe ID card

- ~ 132 Kcal calories per serving
- ~ Easy difficulty
- ~ Serves 8
- ~ Preparation 125 minutes
- ~ Low cost
- ~ 90 minutes for cooking lentils; 20 minutes for preparing meatloaf; 15 minutes for cooking meatloaf + 12 hours for soaking lentils

Ingredients

For the Vegetable Meatloaf

- ~ 1 tablespoon extra virgin olive oil
- ~ 200 g of carrots
- ~ salt
- ~ Organic food: 80 g of breadcrumbs
- ~ 40 g of grated Vegan Cheese
- ~ 125 g of tofu
- ~ 150 ml of soy milk
- ~ Homemade whole food: 150 g of stale bread
- ~ 800 g of boiled lentils or 300 g of dried lentils

For the Vegetable Béchamel

- ~ 1 tablespoon extra virgin olive oil
- ~ 1 grated nutmeg
- ~ pepper
- ~ salt

- ~ 20 g of cornstarch
- ~ 200 ml of soy milk

Material Required

- ~ Bowls of various sizes
- ~ Wooden spoon
- ~ Saucepan
- ~ Oval casserole dish
- ~ Whisk
- ~ Aluminum paper
- ~ Blender

Preparation

First, soak 300 g of dried lentils for 10-12 hours.

Rinse the soaked lentils and cook them in plenty of unsalted water for 90-120 minutes, until soft.

Meanwhile, peel a couple of carrots and boil them for 20 minutes.

Drain the lentils from the cooking water and salt to taste.

Prepare the vegan béchamel sauce: dissolve 20 g of corn-starch in the soy milk. Add salt and pepper and flavor the vegetable milk with nutmeg: cook until boiling, adding a tablespoon of oil. When the béchamel begins to thicken, turn off the heat, stir with a whisk and set aside.

Soften the stale whole-wheat bread in the hot soy milk and squeeze it to remove any excess liquid.

Add the soaked bread, béchamel, salt and vegan grated cheese to the lentils: stir to combine all ingredients. Blend the tofu and add to the mixture.

At this point, add as much breadcrumbs as necessary until soft and slightly sticky.

Spread the mixture on a sheet of aluminium foil, taking care to form a sausage. Gently insert the two carrots in the middle of the dough and, with hands greased with oil, close the meatloaf.

Roll the vegetable meatloaf with aluminium foil. If necessary, use some rubber bands to seal it tighter.

Pour plenty of water into an oval saucepan and bring to a boil. When the water boils, gently add the rolled meatloaf to the aluminium foil and cook for 15 minutes (from the time of boiling).

Remove the meatloaf from the water and allow it to cool completely.

Cut the lentil meatloaf into slices a couple of inches wide. Reheat individual slices and serve with raw vegetables or a tomato sauce.

Pumpkin Mash

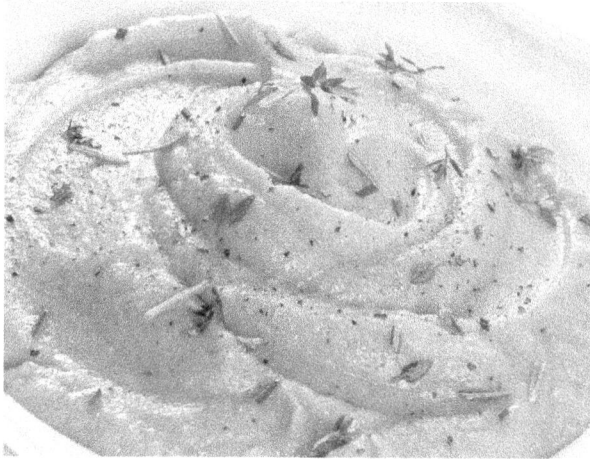

Recipe ID card

- ~ 118 Kcal calories per serving
- ~ Easy difficulty
- ~ Serves 4
- ~ Preparation 20 minutes
- ~ Low cost

Ingredients

- ~ 20 g of grated Parmesan cheese
- ~ about 80-100 ml of milk
- ~ 1 grated nutmeg
- ~ 2 tablespoons of extra virgin olive oil
- ~ 1 pinch of pepper
- ~ 1 sprig of rosemary
- ~ 1 pinch of salt
- ~ 500 g of pumpkin pulp

Material Required

- ~ Pan with lid
- ~ Scoop or wooden spoon
- ~ Blender
- ~ Sharp knife
- ~ Cutting board
- ~ Grater

Preparation

First of all clean the pumpkin well: remove the seeds and the internal filaments, then remove the hard skin.

Cut the pumpkin in very small pieces: in this way, cooking time will be shorter.

Heat a pan, add a drizzle of extra-virgin olive oil and brown the pumpkin on a high flame, without a lid.

Once the pumpkin is browned on all sides (be careful not to burn it!), lower the flame and cover with the lid: continue cooking for about 10 minutes, until the flesh is soft.

A few minutes before the end of cooking, add a pinch of salt, a little pepper, grate in a pinch of nutmeg and flavor with a sprig of rosemary.

Let the pumpkin cool down, then blend it finely until it is reduced to a cream.

Heat the milk in a small saucepan and add it to the pumpkin puree. Stir in a handful of Parmesan cheese and serve as a side dish or use as desired to make tortellini, bread and pies.

Topinambur Trifoliated

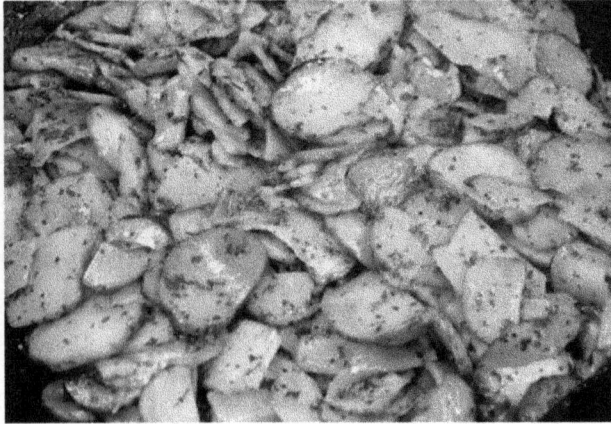

Recipe ID card

- ~ 102 Kcal calories per serving
- ~ Easy difficulty
- ~ Serves 4
- ~ Preparation 15 minutes
- ~ Low cost
- ~ 15 minutes for preparation; 15 minutes for cooking

Ingredients

- ~ 700 g of Jerusalem artichokes
- ~ 2-3 spoons of dry white wine
- ~ 1 garlic clove
- ~ 1 tuft of parsley
- ~ Peel of untreated lemon
- ~ 2 spoons of extra virgin olive oil
- ~ salt
- ~ pepper
- ~ If necessary: 50 ml of vegetable broth or water

Material Required

- ~ Knife
- ~ Bowl
- ~ Latex gloves (optional)
- ~ Grater (for lemon zest)
- ~ Cutting board
- ~ Knife
- ~ Pan with lid

Preparation

Wash the Jerusalem artichokes well in running water, possibly scrubbing them with a brush to remove impurities and traces of soil.

Dry the Jerusalem artichokes and cut them into slices with the help of a simple knife.

As you cut, dip the Jerusalem artichoke slices into a solution of water and lemon juice.

Pour 2 tablespoons of e.v.o. oil into an already very hot pan and flavor with a clove of garlic. Those who like the taste of garlic can crush the pulp directly in the oil; those who do not like it particularly, can brown the whole clove in the oil and remove it after a few minutes.

Drain the Jerusalem artichokes from the acidulated water and pour them into the flavoured oil. Sauté over high heat.

Season with salt and pepper to taste. Deglaze with the white wine, cover the pan with the lid and cook over moderate heat for 20-25 minutes, stirring occasionally.

Should the Jerusalem artichokes be excessively dry, it is advisable to add half a glass of hot water or vegetable broth while cooking.

At the end of cooking, the Jerusalem artichokes should appear firm, but not crunchy. Therefore turn off the flame and season with abundant chopped parsley and lemon zest.

Bread, Pizza and Brioche for Diabetics

Brioches with wholemeal flour

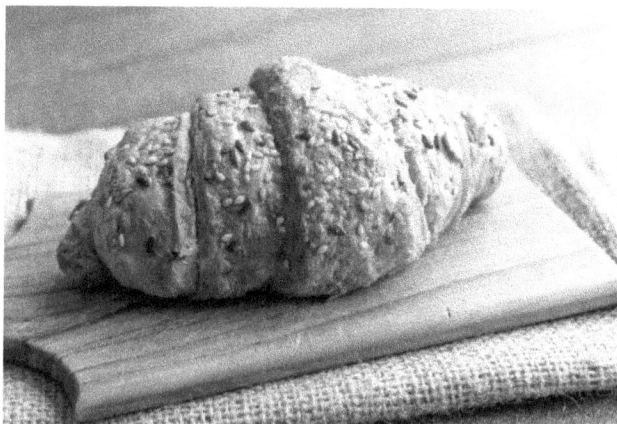

Recipe ID card

- ~ 273 Kcal calories per serving
- ~ Difficulty fairly easy
- ~ Serves 8
- ~ Preparation 50 minutes
- ~ Low cost
- ~ 20 minutes to prepare + 10 hours to rise (6 hours for the leavening + 3 hours for the first rise + 1 hour for the second rise) + 20 minutes to bake

Ingredients

To decorate

- ~ a sprinkling of icing sugar

For the leaven

- ~ 110 g of Manitoba flour
- ~ 80 ml of water
- ~ 20 g of brewer's yeast
- ~ 5 g of honey

For the filling

- ~ 100 g of jam

For the main dough

- ~ 60 g of butter
- ~ 40 ml of water
- ~ 70 g of honey
- ~ grated rind of untreated lemon
- ~ 1 pinch of salt
- ~ 60 g (1 medium) of eggs
- ~ 190 g of Manitoba flour
- ~ 120 g of wholemeal flour

Material Required

- ~ Bowls of various sizes
- ~ Film
- ~ Wooden ladles
- ~ Sharp knife or wheel
- ~ Brush
- ~ Baking paper
- ~ Baking sheets
- ~ Matter
- ~ Spoons
- ~ Pastry board
- ~ Latex gloves (optional)

Preparation

Prepare the yeast (or biga) by dissolving the brewer's yeast in warm water, sweetened with a teaspoon of honey. Mix the dissolved yeast with the Manitoba flour with a wooden spoon until the mixture is very soft and sticky. Let the dough rest overnight, well covered with plastic wrap.

When the dough has swollen, add the remaining Manitoba flour, whole wheat flour, salt (possibly avoiding direct contact with the dough), honey, melted butter and egg. Flavor everything with the grated zest of a lemon or a flavor to taste. You will probably need to add 30-40 ml of water to make the dough soft and smooth (the amount of water depends on the type of whole wheat flour used). Knead the dough for a long time in order to facilitate the formation of gluten: let it rest in a glass bowl for a couple of hours, until the dough has doubled in volume.

When it is puffy and soft, divide the dough into two parts and cut out 2 discs with the help of a rolling pin.

Cut each disc into 8 segments: pour a teaspoon of jam on the base of each triangle obtained. Wrap each triangle on itself, starting from the base, trying to trap the jam in the dough by pressing it with your fingers to prevent it from coming out during the next rising or baking.

Arrange the brioches on two baking sheets lined with parchment paper, taking care to keep a certain distance between them to prevent them from swelling and sticking together. Let rise again until doubled in volume: it will take about an hour.

Once doubled in volume, you can proceed with the baking of the brioches: bake the cakes at 180 ° C and cook for 15 minutes.

Let them cool down and sprinkle with a little powdered sugar to taste.

Wholewheat crackers

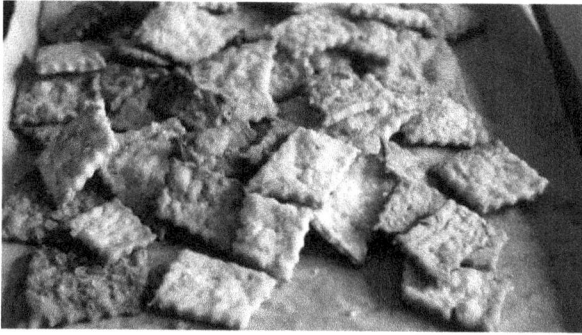

Recipe ID card

~ 264 Kcal calories per serving
~ Easy difficulty
~ Serves 8
~ Preparation 30 minutes
~ Low cost
~ 15 minutes for preparation; 15 minutes for cooking

Ingredients

For the main dough

~ 1 teaspoon of salt
~ chopped rosemary or a sprig of rosemary
~ 2 tablespoons extra virgin olive oil
~ 125 ml of milk
~ 10 g of potato starch
~ 125 g of whole wheat flour
~ 60 g of wheat bran
~ 5 g of ammonium bicarbonate

To brush

~ a pinch of salt
~ 1 tablespoon of extra virgin olive oil
~ about 30 ml of water

Material Required

~ Capacious bowls
~ Wooden ladle
~ Latex gloves (optional)
~ Dough rolling machine or rolling pin
~ 8 cm diameter cookie mold
~ 2 baking sheets
~ Baking paper
~ Brush
~ Small bowl
~ Fork

Preparation

In a large bowl pour the whole wheat flour, wheat bran (or oat bran), salt, potato starch, chopped rosemary and bicarbonate of ammonium.

Once the "powders" are mixed, add the milk (or water) and a couple of tablespoons of extra virgin olive oil. Amalgamate everything with hands and knead the dough for a long time: the consistency of the dough must be similar to that of traditional bread.

At this point, divide the dough into two parts and roll it out very finely with a rolling pin or a pasta machine: a 2-3 mm thick sheet should be obtained.

With a round-shaped cookie cutter, cut out many crackers from the dough sheets obtained. The scraps can be kneaded again to form more crackers.

Place the discs of dough on two baking sheets previously lined with greaseproof paper. Prick the crackers with a fork to prevent them from swelling excessively during cooking.

In a small bowl, pour a little water and a drop of extra virgin olive oil: emulsify everything and brush this liquid on the surface of each crackers. Those who wish can sprinkle each disc with a little fine salt.

Bake the crackers at 200°C for about 10-15 minutes, until crispy.

Immediately remove the crackers from the plates and let them cool completely on a wire rack. Once cooled, store the crackers in an airtight container.

Rustic loaf with carrots

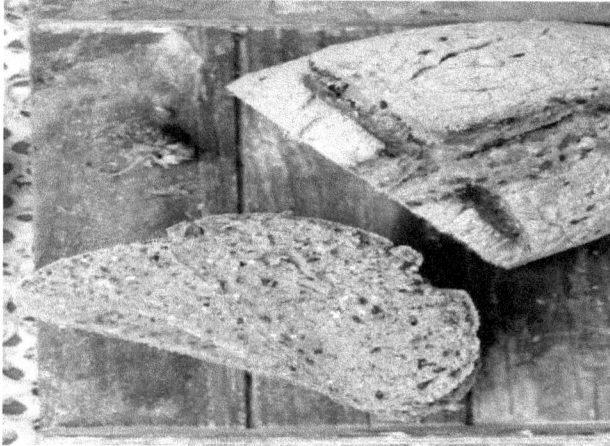

- ~ Electric or manual grater for carrots
- ~ Vegetable peeler for carrots

Preparation

Wash, dry and peel the carrots. Grate them in the electric (or manual) grater until you get many thin sticks.

Crumble the brewer's yeast in a glass, add the sugar (to activate the yeast) and dissolve it by adding a little warm water. Stir with a wooden stick (avoid steel) to avoid compromising yeast fermentation.

In a bowl, pour the flour and, in the center, add the yeast dissolved in the water. Then add salt, being very careful to avoid direct contact between salt and yeast. At this point, add the remaining part of warm water and the carrots.

Knead vigorously and for a long time in order to promote the formation of gluten during baking: this will result in a very soft bread.

Transfer the ball of dough into a round mold with a diameter of 18 cm, without adding oil. Let rest for about an hour (or until doubled in volume) in a warm place.

Bake the pan in a hot, preheated oven at a high temperature (220°C) for 15 minutes. After this period, without opening the oven door, lower the temperature to 190°C and continue cooking for another 15-20 minutes.

Allow to cool before cutting the loaf.

Recipe ID card

- ~ 173 Kcal calories per serving
- ~ Easy difficulty
- ~ Serves 6
- ~ Preparation 105 minutes
- ~ Low cost
- ~ 10 minutes for dough; 60 minutes for rising; 35 minutes for baking

Ingredients

- ~ 400 g of Manitoba flour
- ~ 200 ml of water
- ~ 160 g (julienned) carrots
- ~ 9 g of salt
- ~ 5 g of sugar
- ~ 20 g of brewer's yeast

Material Required

- ~ Hinged baking pan with a diameter of 18 cm
- ~ Pastry board
- ~ Wooden stick
- ~ Glass
- ~ Large bowl
- ~ Latex gloves (optional)
- ~ Flour bowl
- ~ Wooden ladle

Wholemeal Bread

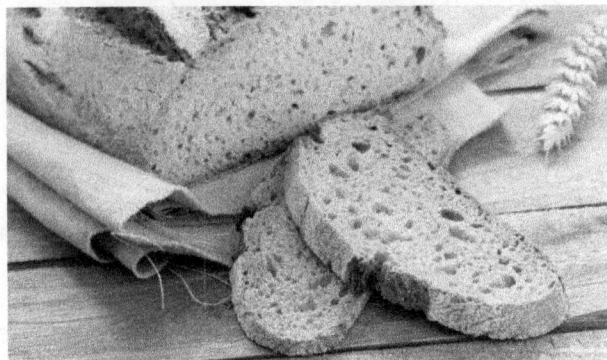

Recipe ID card

- ~ 226 Kcal calories per serving
- ~ Difficulty fairly easy
- ~ Serves 4
- ~ Preparation 320 minutes
- ~ Low cost
- ~ 30 minutes + 4.5 hours rising time + 20 minutes baking time

Ingredients

For the leaven

- ~ 100 g of whole wheat flour
- ~ 100 ml water
- ~ 10 g of brewer's yeast
- ~ 1 teaspoon of brown sugar

For the main dough

- ~ 400 g whole wheat flour
- ~ 12 g of salt
- ~ 2 tablespoons of extra virgin olive oil
- ~ 200 ml of water

Material Required

- ~ Bowls
- ~ Pastry board
- ~ Wooden spoon
- ~ Transparent film
- ~ Food scale
- ~ Baking tray
- ~ Baking paper
- ~ Rolling pin
- ~ Knife or pizza wheel

Preparation

First prepare the leaven by mixing the whole wheat flour with the brewer's yeast dissolved in water softened with brown sugar: a thick batter should be formed.

Cover the bowl with plastic wrap and leave to rise for an hour until surface bubbles form.

Now prepare the main dough by mixing the remaining whole-wheat flour with the oil, water and salt. Add the yeast (which will have taken on a swollen and foamy consistency) and knead the dough vigorously with your hands.

Place the dough back in the bowl and cover with plastic wrap. Let rise 3 hours or until the dough has tripled in volume.

Remove the puffy dough from the bowl and roll it out on the pastry board with the help of a rolling pin, until it forms a rectangle with approximate dimensions of 30X40 cm.

From the rectangular sheet obtain 8 strips of dough: wrap each strip around itself, taking care not to overtighten it.

Place each roll on the baking sheet, with the end facing down to prevent it from opening during rising or baking.

Let rise again for 40-60 minutes until the buns are puffy.

Bake in a static oven, preheated to 200°C, for 20-25 minutes.

Let cool on a wire rack and serve.

Whole wheat pizza

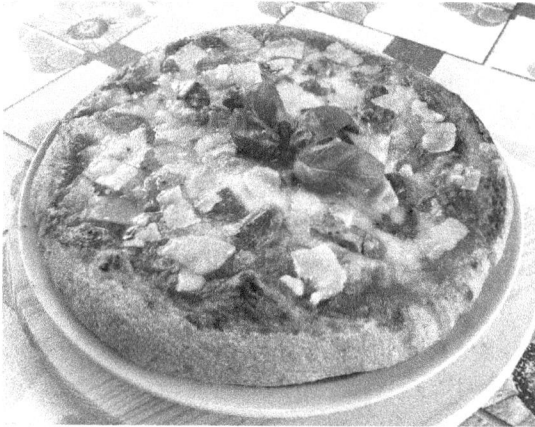

Recipe ID card

~ 160 Kcal calories per serving
~ Difficulty fairly easy
~ Serves 4
~ Preparation 20 minutes
~ Low cost
~ 10 minutes for preparation; 36 hours rest; 10 minutes for cooking

Ingredients

For the pasta

~ 200 g of whole wheat flour
~ 180 g of Manitoba flour
~ 3 g fresh brewer's yeast or 1 g dried brewer's yeast
~ 9 g of salt
~ 220 ml water

For the filling

~ 200 g of cherry tomatoes
~ A few basil leaves
~ 250 g of mozzarella
~ 200 g of tomato puree
~ 1 bunch of rocket

Material Required

~ Baking stone plate or baking sheet
~ Baking shovel
~ Bowl
~ Baking paper
~ Cling film
~ Chopping board or pastry board

Preparation

In a bowl, combine the Manitoba flour and whole wheat flour. Mix the powders with the dry brewer's yeast, then add the salt and mix with enough water (about 220 ml) to obtain a soft and elastic dough.

Grease the bowl with a little oil, then place the dough inside and cover with plastic wrap. Let the dough rest at room temperature for an hour. Then put the bowl in the fridge and let it rest for 24-36 hours.

After 36 hours have passed, remove the bowl from the fridge and let the dough sit at room temperature for an hour.

Cut the dough into two parts. Roll out the dough with hands until obtaining two discs as regular as possible; if necessary, spread a layer of flour on the working surface. The use of a rolling pin is not recommended.

Preheat the oven to the maximum temperature (250-280°C), taking care to place the refractory stone plate on the base.

Stuff one pizza disc at a time with tomato puree, mozzarella and cherry tomatoes.

Remove the pizza with the special shovel and place it on the stone baking tray. Cook for 8-10 minutes, according to the characteristics of your oven.

Remove the pizza from the oven using the shovel and finish with fresh basil and arugula. Repeat the operation with the other disc of dough.

Gluten Free Pizza with Pea Flour

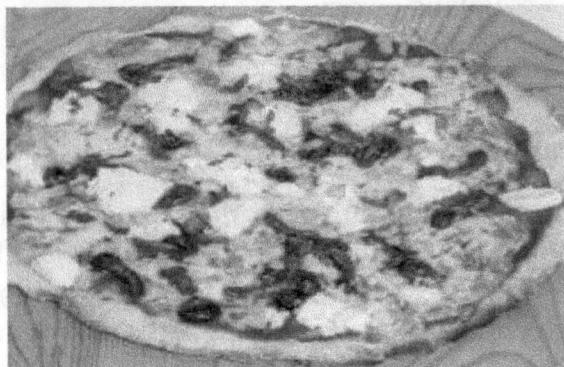

Recipe ID card

- ~ 190 Kcal calories per serving
- ~ Easy difficulty
- ~ Serves 2
- ~ Preparation 125 minutes
- ~ Low cost
- ~ 15 minutes for preparation; 90 minutes for rising; 20 minutes for baking

Ingredients

For the dough

- ~ 150 g of pea flour
- ~ 3 tablespoons of extra virgin olive oil
- ~ 165 ml of water
- ~ 5 g of sugar
- ~ 10 g of brewer's yeast
- ~ 8 g of salt
- ~ 45 g of rice flour
- ~ 80 g of cornstarch

For the filling

- ~ Ready-made: 100 g artichokes
- ~ 125 g of mozzarella
- ~ 100 g of tomato puree

Material Required

- ~ Bowl
- ~ Transparent film
- ~ Glass
- ~ Stick
- ~ Sieve
- ~ Cheese blender (optional)
- ~ Baking tray
- ~ Baking paper

Preparation

In a bowl, sift pea flour, cornmeal and rice flour.

Dissolve the sugar in 100 ml warm water. Crumble the brewer's yeast into the warm water and stir with a wooden stick.

Pour the yeast dissolved in the water into the center of the flours and let it rest about 15-20 minutes, until the yeast has become puffy and soft.

At this point, add the remaining water, salt and 2 tablespoons of extra virgin olive oil: mix well until the dough is soft and not sticky.

Line a baking pan with baking paper.

Grease the baking sheet with a tablespoon of oil and place the ball of dough on it: crush the dough with your hands, turning it to distribute the oil evenly and to make it easier to roll out. A disc of dough half a centimetre thick should be obtained.

Leave the dough to rise in a warm place for about an hour, until it has puffed up.

Spread the tomato puree over the surface of the pizza and bake in a preheated oven at 180°C for 10 minutes.

Meanwhile, blend the cheese or cut it into small pieces with a knife.

After 10 minutes, remove the pizza from the oven and top with the shredded mozzarella and a few artichokes.

Bake again and finish cooking for another 10 minutes.

Vegan Pizza with Algae and Vegetable Cheese

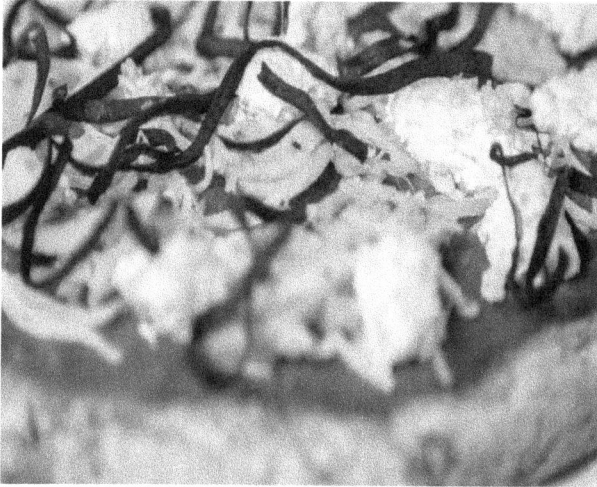

Recipe ID card

- ~ Easy difficulty
- ~ Serves 2
- ~ Preparation 40 minutes
- ~ Average cost
- ~ 15 minutes for preparation; 25 minutes for cooking

Ingredients

For the dough

- ~ 150 g of wholemeal flour
- ~ 2 tablespoons of extra virgin olive oil
- ~ 5 g of salt
- ~ 8 g of instant yeast
- ~ 240 ml of vegetable ricotta whey or 240 ml of water
- ~ 80 g of soy flour

For the filling

- ~ 100 g of tomato puree
- ~ 50 g of fresh ricotta cheese
- ~ 50 g of vegetable cheese
- ~ 4 g of spaghetti seaweed
- ~ 50 g of soybean sprouts

Material Required

- ~ Bowl
- ~ Wooden spoon
- ~ 28 cm diameter baking dish
- ~ Sieve
- ~ Food scale
- ~ Dish

Preparation

First, soak the spaghetti seaweed in warm water.

Preheat the oven to 180 °C.

In a bowl, mix the whole wheat flour with the soy flour. Then add the sieved instant yeast and salt.

In the center, add the liquids, or the whey of vegetable ricotta (or plain water) and a tablespoon of olive oil.

Knead thoroughly until you get a soft and mouldable dough.

Pour a tablespoon of oil in a baking pan with a diameter of 28 cm; distribute the dough, pressing it with your hands. Stuff the dough with the tomato puree.

Bake the pizza with the tomato base in a preheated oven and bake for 15 minutes.

Remove the pizza from the oven and stuff to taste with slices of pea vegetable cheese, clumps of vegetable ricotta, the soy sprouts and the spaghetti seaweed (well squeezed out of the soaking water).

Finish baking in the oven for an additional 10 minutes.

Sandwich Light

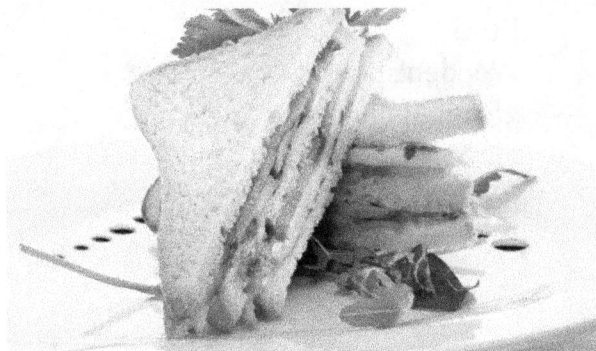

Preparation

Spread 50 g of ricotta cheese on a slice of rye bread (each slice of bread weighs 60 g).

Wash the tomato and cut it into very thin slices. Place the tomato slices on top of the ricotta.

Wash a few green salad leaves. Arrange the leaves on top of the tomato.

At this point prepare the filling of the second layer. Prepare the eggless mayonnaise.

Prepare the parmesan cheese flakes using a vegetable peeler.

Cut the gherkins into thin slices.

Spread a second slice of rye bread with 15 g of egg-free mayonnaise. Arrange the bresaola slices on top of the mayonnaise; add the grana cheese flakes and the gherkin slices.

Spread the remaining ricotta on the third slice of rye bread.

Compose the sandwich, taking care to turn the slice with the ricotta towards the filling.

Let the sandwich rest in the fridge for an hour or so.

Recipe ID card

~ 121 Kcal calories per serving
~ Easy difficulty
~ Serves 4
~ Preparation 15 minutes
~ Low cost
~ 15 minutes + 1 hour cooling time

Ingredients

~ 3 slices (180 g) of rye bread or sandwich bread
~ 70 g of fresh ricotta cheese
~ 80 g of coppery tomatoes
~ A few leaves of tender salad
~ 50 g of bresaola
~ 10 g of grated parmesan cheese
~ 30 g of gherkins
~ 15 g of vegan mayonnaise or light mayonnaise or yoghurt mayonnaise

Material Required

~ Cutting board
~ Knives
~ Food scale
~ Sandwich sticks
~ Vegetable peeler (for flakes)
~ Dipping mixer for mayonnaise

Basic Preparations for Diabetics

Watermelon

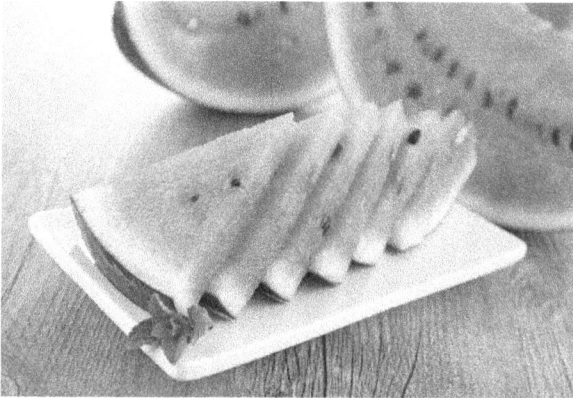

Recipe ID card

~ 33 Kcal calories per serving
~ Difficulty fairly easy
~ Serves 4
~ Preparation 15 minutes
~ Low cost

Ingredients

~ 5 kg of watermelon

Material Required

~ Watermelon slicer
~ Long blade knife
~ Digger

Preparation

CLASSIC WATERMELON CUTTING. Wash the watermelon to remove any traces of soil and dirt. Lay the watermelon horizontally on a plane: with a knife, cut the part of the stem and the opposite side so as to create two smooth surfaces. Now, arrange the fruit vertically, resting one of the two cut sides directly on the work surface. Using a long-bladed knife, cut the watermelon in half, taking care to create two equal parts. Cut the watermelon into wedges (lengthwise); run a short-bladed knife along the flesh, so as to separate the red part from the white part. Once sliced, cut the flesh into triangles. Serve the watermelon triangles directly on the peel, alternating the slices to create a boat (same presentation you use to serve pineapple). This method is best for small watermelons (baby watermelons) and medium-sized round watermelons.

CUTTING WITH WATERMELON SLICER. Wash the watermelon to remove soil and dirt. Lay the watermelon horizontally on a plane and cut it in half to obtain two equal sections. Insert the appropriate tool (watermelon slicer) with the curved part facing upwards, inside the pulp, near the narrowest part of the fruit: pushing the tool in depth, draw the slice. Remove the tool and repeat the operation until the opposite end of the fruit is reached. At this point, turn the tool in order to have the curved part facing downwards: introduce the tool and, by using it as if it were pliers, take the slice and serve it on a plate. This method is suitable for serving all types of watermelon.

CUTTING WITH THE DIGGER. After having washed and cut watermelon in half, it is possible to dig the pulp with a small digger in order to obtain many small balls, as we have seen in the preparation of melon. Watermelon balls are very beautiful to see and convenient to serve, perfect for fruit salads, skewers or cocktails.

CUT INTO SMALL SLICES (WITH PEEL). Wash watermelon and cut in half to make two equal sections. Place one half on the work surface, leaning the pulp down. Taking care, cut the peel first, then cut the pulp too and obtain regular slices 2-3 cm wide: it is advisable to start from the part of the stalk towards the opposite part. At pleasure, slices can be cut in half or in quarters. This method is ideal for oval watermelons.

PEEL THE WATERMELON COMPLETELY. Wash the watermelon and cut it in half to make two equal sections. Place one half on the work surface, resting the flesh down. Using a sharp knife, remove the skin from the watermelon, taking care to remove the green part and the white part. Cut the watermelon flesh into slices to make crescents or smaller pieces. This method is adaptable to any type of watermelon.

How to Open and Clean the Coconut

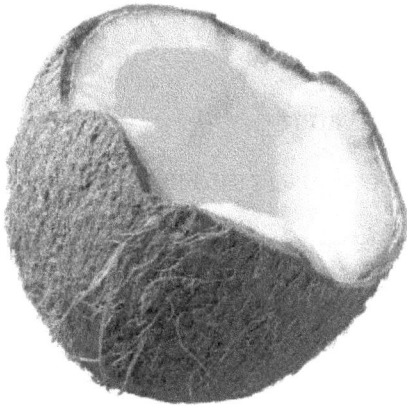

Recipe ID card

~ 364 Kcal calories per serving
~ Difficult difficulty
~ Serves 6
~ Preparation 15 minutes
~ Low cost

Ingredients

~ 1 coconut

Material Required

~ Dishcloth
~ Hammer
~ Screwdriver, corkscrew or other sharp object
~ Glass
~ Colander
~ Sterile gauze or strong absorbent paper
~ Transparent film for storage
~ Bowl

Preparation

Using a corkscrew, pierce two of the three eyes located in one end of the coconut.

Turn the coconut upside down and let all the liquid (called "coconut water") come out.

Then proceed with the breaking of the coconut: with a hammer, tap the coconut while turning it around. The blows must be rather firm: the coconut will easily break.

To break the pieces obtained in smaller parts, proceed with more hammer blows.

With a knife, remove the pulp from the shell by exerting some pressure, then wash the pieces in cold water.

For preservation, it is recommended to soak coconut pieces in the same liquid extracted from the nut. Alternatively, cover the coconut with fresh water and keep in the fridge (change the water every day) for 3-4 days.

How to Clean and Cook Thistles

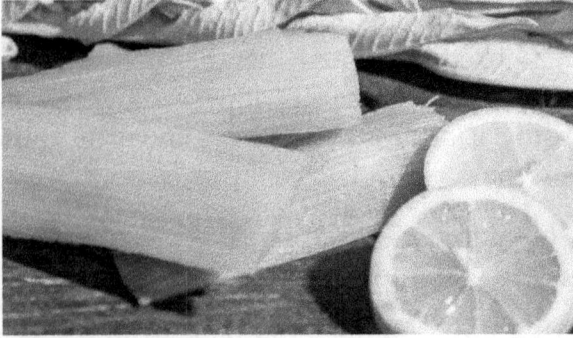

Recipe ID card

~ 155 Kcal calories per serving
~ Easy difficulty
~ Serves 6
~ Preparation 20 minutes
~ Low cost
~ 20 minutes for cleaning; about 1 hour for boiling

Ingredients

~ 6 long ribs (500 g, clean weight) of cardoons
~ 100 g of untreated lemon
~ water
~ salt

Material Required

~ Bowl
~ Vegetable peeler or knife
~ Cutting board
~ Casserole
~ Latex gloves (optional)
~ Casserole

Preparation

Prepare a bowl with water and lemon juice.

Separate the ribs from the head, removing any leaves. Cut the stalks into pieces about 10 cm long and, if they are particularly large or wide, cut them lengthwise as well.

Remove the hard, woody filaments from each piece of rib using a sharp knife or a vegetable peeler (recommended). As the ribs are cleaned, plunge the cardoons into the acidulated water.

Rinse the cardoons under running water.

Boil a saucepan full of water. When the water boils, add a little salt and add the cardoons: cook for about an hour or until soft.

Drain the ribs of the cardoons from the water and cover with plastic wrap. The cardoons are ready to be seasoned at will: they can be sautéed in a pan with oil, garlic and parsley, fried in oil or baked au gratin with béchamel sauce. Cardoons are excellent for the realization of savoury pies and soups.

How to Clean and Cook Octopus

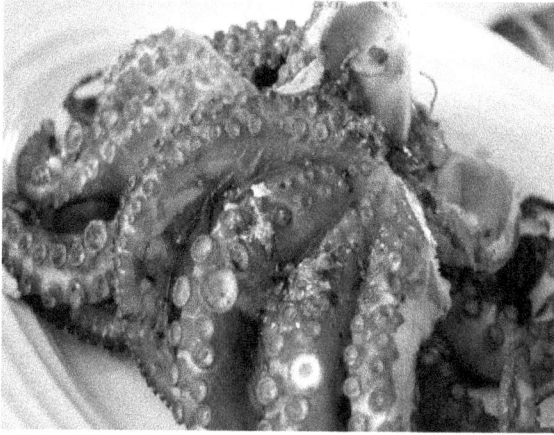

Recipe ID card

- ~ 74 Kcal calories per serving
- ~ Difficulty fairly easy
- ~ Serves 4
- ~ Preparation 15 minutes
- ~ Average cost
- ~ 15 minutes for cleaning; 20 minutes (+ cooling time) for cooking

Ingredients

- ~ 1 Kg of octopus
- ~ 100 g of carrots
- ~ Untreated lemon juice
- ~ 2 celery stalks
- ~ salt
- ~ water

Material Required

- ~ Cutting board
- ~ Meat tenderizer or food hammer
- ~ Very large saucepan
- ~ Knife
- ~ Fork
- ~ Blotting paper

Preparation

If the octopus is fresh, the first thing to do is to cut into the base of the body bag without separating it from the tentacles, turning it upside down to remove the entrails. Thawed octopus are already eviscerated.

Remove the eyes of the octopus by making an incision.

Then make an incision in the tooth (rostrum) and remove it by pushing it with your fingers.

Roll the meat to break the fibres and tenderize it: then gently beat the head and tentacles with a meat pounder. In this way, the octopus meat will be tender and not rubbery.

Wash the octopus in running water, insisting on the suckers to remove any impurities.

The octopus can now be cooked or frozen.

Boil plenty of water and flavor with celery, carrot and lemon juice. Salt to taste. Those who wish can also add an onion.

When the water boils, immerse and quickly extract the tentacles 6-7 times, lifting it by the head: in this way the tentacles will curl and the meat will be more tender.

Immerse the octopus and calculate 20 minutes per kilo of mollusc: the octopus should boil very gently. After the necessary time has elapsed, turn off the fire and allow to cool completely in the cooking water.

Once it has reached room temperature, the octopus can be removed from the water. By piercing the cooked octopus with a fork, it will be possible to perceive the softness of the flesh.

Those who wish can scrape the skin off the tentacles for a better presentation of the boiled octopus.

The octopus can be cut in more or less regular pieces and used immediately to prepare salads or it can be frozen (in pieces) and kept for 2-3 months.

How to Clean and Cut Pumpkin

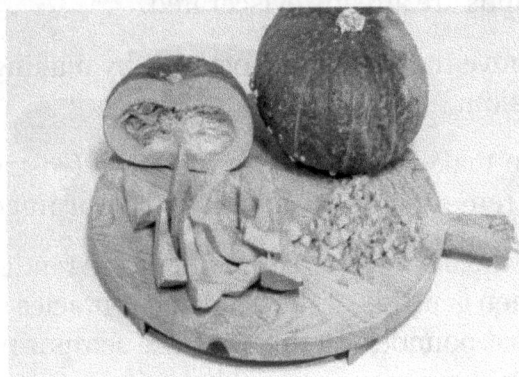

Recipe ID card

~ 18 Kcal calories per serving
~ Difficult difficulty
~ Serves 8 people
~ Preparation 15 minutes
~ Low cost

Ingredients

~ 2 kg (1 medium) of pumpkin

Material Required

~ Knives of different sizes
~ 1 digger or 1 steel spoon
~ 1 chopping board or wooden board
~ Brush (optional)

Preparation

First of all, wash the pumpkin very well in fresh water, rubbing off any traces of soil. It can be made easier by using a small brush.

Using a sharp knife with a long blade, cut the pumpkin in half. In case the pumpkin is very large, it is advisable to cut the peel with the knife and run it along the whole diameter of the pumpkin, until it is cut in half.

Using a small digger or a simple steel spoon, remove the internal filaments and seeds.

Cut the pumpkin in quarters and in eighths: the smaller the pieces are, the easier it will be to remove the external peel.

In order to remove the rind it is advisable to use a long blade knife. Place the base of each piece of pumpkin on a cutting board and hold the piece firmly with one hand, keeping the fingers as far as possible from the base. With the other hand, cut the rind and slide the knife up to the cutting board: cuts must be clean and firm. Turn the piece of pumpkin over and repeat the operation from the opposite side.

Cut the pumpkin in slices or in smaller squares, according to the use. Cook the pumpkin as desired: it is ready when the inside is very soft.

How to Clean Eggplants

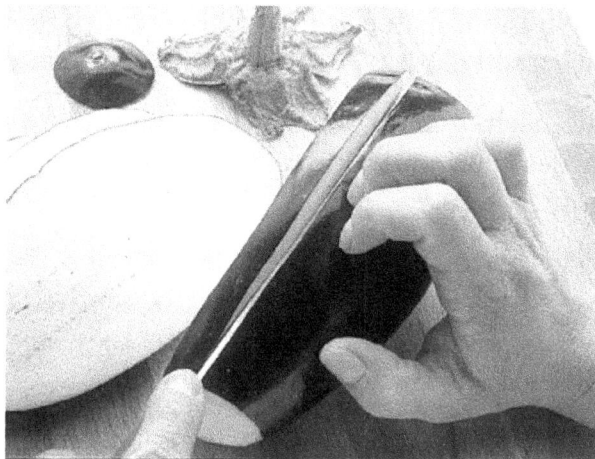

Place a strainer or colander over a plate or bowl, then gather the eggplant slices, sprinkling with coarse salt as you go.

Let the eggplants drip for a couple of hours: to facilitate the dripping, it is advisable to put a weight on top of the eggplants.

When the liquid has collected in the bowl, wash the eggplants in water to remove any traces of salt and gently squeeze them to remove the water.

Eggplants are ready to be cooked in a variety of ways: they can be tossed in paella with oil and spices (e.g. eggplant mushrooms), breaded and cooked in the oven or in oil (eggplant cutlets), blended to make sauces or purees, grilled or cooked on the grill to make eggplant rolls, Parmigiana or much more.

Recipe ID card

~ 27 Kcal calories per serving
~ Easy difficulty
~ Serves 4
~ Preparation 20 minutes
~ Low cost
~ 20 minutes for preparation; 2 hours for draining

Ingredients

For the salt treatment

~ 700 g (2 medium-sized) eggplants
~ 1 tablespoon of coarse salt

Material Required

~ Cutting board
~ Knife
~ Pasta drainer
~ Bowl

Preparation

Wash the eggplants, trim them to remove the stalk and cut them into 1 cm thick slices (or into cubes). If desired, you can peel them.

Classic Tomato Conserve

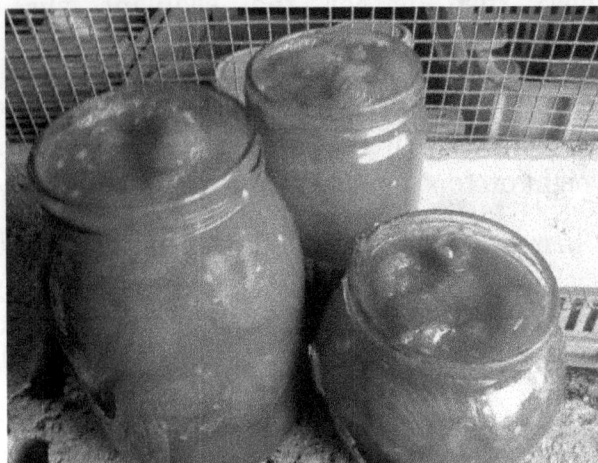

Recipe ID card

~ 17 Kcal calories per serving
~ Difficulty quite easy
~ Serves 10 people
~ Preparation 60 minutes
~ Low cost

Ingredients

~ 2 Kg of San Marzano tomatoes
~ Optional: a few basil leaves

Material Required

~ Large saucepan
~ Chopping board
~ Knife
~ Vegetable mill
~ Glass jars with respective screw caps
~ Sponge
~ Tea towels
~ Latex gloves (optional)
~ Wooden ladles and spoons
~ Pasta strainer (optional)
~ Large bowls
~ Tongs
~ Funnel

Preparation

Wash the tomatoes thoroughly and dry them with a soft cloth.

Cut each tomato lengthwise, removing the hardest part and the seeds with the help of a knife.

Pour the tomatoes into a saucepan and cook over very gentle heat, stirring frequently. The tomatoes will be ready when they have softened and formed almost a mush.

Meanwhile, in a very large saucepan filled with water, boil the glass jars with their respective screw caps.

Pass the tomatoes through a vegetable mill and collect the resulting conserve. If it is excessively liquid, filter it again through a clean cloth and collect only the pulp.

Pour the tomato pulp back into the saucepan and bring to a boil.

Remove the sterilized jars and caps from the water and, immediately, fill the jars with the tomato puree while still boiling, leaving at least 2 cm from the top edge. Those who wish can add some basil leaves directly into the jar.

Close the jars with the caps and let them cool down: by potting the tomato puree while it is still boiling (on freshly sterilized and equally boiling jars), it will not be necessary to follow the instructions for the classic post-potting sterilization.

Homemade Curry

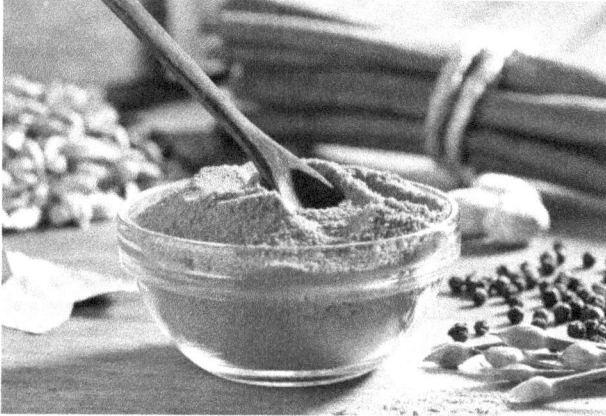

them to powder with the help of a pestle. Mix the obtained powder with turmeric powder.

You can modulate the flavor by adding other spices such as: nutmeg, hot pepper, cardamom, fenugreek, ginger, mace, anise, garlic etc.

Collect curry in a jar with screw cap and store in a dry place, away from light. Consume within a couple of months.

Recipe ID card

~ 342 Kcal calories per serving
~ Easy difficulty
~ Serves 20
~ Preparation 10 minutes
~ Low cost

Ingredients

~ 1 tablespoon turmeric powder
~ 1 teaspoon of cumin seeds
~ 1 teaspoon of fennel seeds
~ 1/4 teaspoon of coriander seeds
~ 2 pieces of cloves
~ 1 piece of cinnamon
~ 4 peppercorns
~ 1 teaspoon mustard seeds

Material Required

~ Mortar with pestle
~ Jar with screw cap

Preparation

Place the spices (coriander seeds, cumin seeds, fennel seeds, cloves, cinnamon, black pepper and mustard seeds) in a mortar and reduce

Homemade Coconut Milk

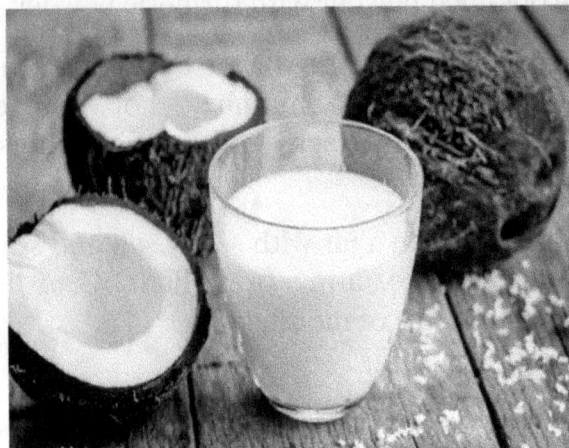

Recipe ID card

- ~ Difficulty quite easy
- ~ Serves 4
- ~ Preparation 30 minutes
- ~ Low cost
- ~ 10 minutes for preparation + 20 minutes for maceration

Ingredients

Proportions to be respected to prepare coconut milk

- ~ 2 parts (e.g. 1.6L) water
- ~ 1 part grated pulp (e.g. 300g) of coconut

Material Required

- ~ Manual or electric grater
- ~ Beaker blender
- ~ Clean dishcloth
- ~ Pasta strainer
- ~ Bowl
- ~ Bottle or jars
- ~ Corkscrew or screwdriver
- ~ Hammer
- ~ Glass

Preparation

First, remove the water naturally present in the coconut: pierce the coconut with a screwdriver or corkscrew. Turn the nut upside down on a glass to extract all the coconut water.

Break the coconut with the help of a hammer and remove the pulp from the hard, woody rind. Watch the fun video on breaking up coconut.

Grate the coconut pulp with an electric or hand grater: continue grating until a cup is filled.

Fill two cups (of equal capacity) with water. Pour water into a small saucepan and heat until almost boiling.

Pour the grated coconut pulp into a blender cup and add the very hot water. Mix intermittently for a couple of minutes. Allow the coconut to macerate 20 minutes: this will promote the extraction of nutrients from the coconut.

Strain through a clean tea towel and wring out to remove all of the vegetation milk.

Bottle or jar the coconut milk and keep in the refrigerator for 2-3 days.

It is always recommended to mix the product before consuming it because coconut milk, being rich in fats, will undergo a natural phase separation.

Light Mayonnaise Without Oil

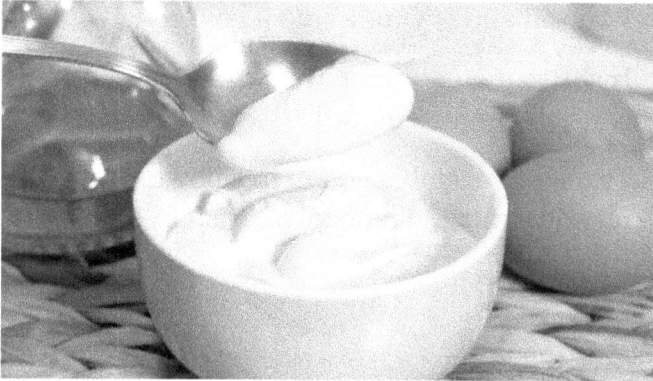

Recipe ID card

- ~ 49 Kcal calories per serving
- ~ Easy difficulty
- ~ Serves 6
- ~ Preparation 10 minutes
- ~ Low cost
- ~ 10 minutes + cooling time (about 1 hour)

Ingredients

- ~ 180 ml of water
- ~ 14 g rice flour
- ~ 20 g (1 medium) of egg yolks
- ~ 1 pinch of salt
- ~ 1 tablespoon untreated lemon juice
- ~ 5 ml vinegar
- ~ half a teaspoon of mustard

Material Required

- ~ Saucepan
- ~ Whisk
- ~ Bowl
- ~ Glass
- ~ Spoon
- ~ Colander

Preparation

Heat about 150 m of water together with a pinch of salt and the mustard.

Pour the rice flour into a glass and add the remaining water (about 30 ml): stir everything together with a teaspoon.

As soon as the water in the saucepan begins to boil, pour in the rice flour and continue stirring with a whisk until a thick cream forms.

Lower the heat and add the lemon juice, vinegar and, last of all, the egg yolk: continue stirring until the desired density is reached.

Pour the cream obtained into a small bowl and leave to cool, first at room temperature, then in the refrigerator.

Homemade Vegetable Cream

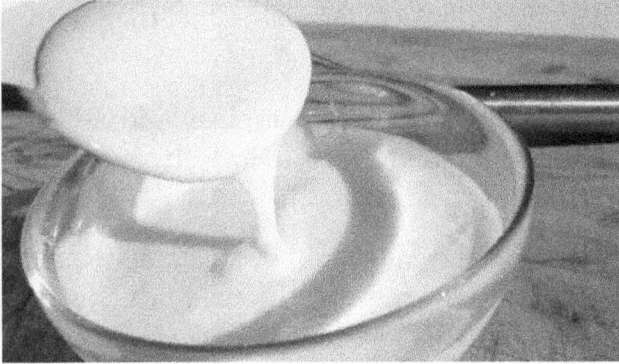

Preparation

Pour oil and soy milk into a beaker.

Insert mixer and blend until desired consistency is achieved.

Transfer vegetable cream to a bowl, cover with plastic wrap and let cool at least an hour.

Recipe ID card

~ 570 Kcal calories per serving
~ Difficulty very easy
~ Serves 6
~ Preparation 5 minutes
~ Low cost
~ 5 minutes + cooling time (about 1 hour)

Ingredients

~ Proportions to be respected to obtain a thick and creamy vegetable cream:
~ 1 part (100 ml) soy milk
~ 2 parts (about 180 ml) of corn oil

Material Required

~ Immersion Mixer
~ Becker or high-sided container
~ Spatula
~ Bowl

Tomato Puree

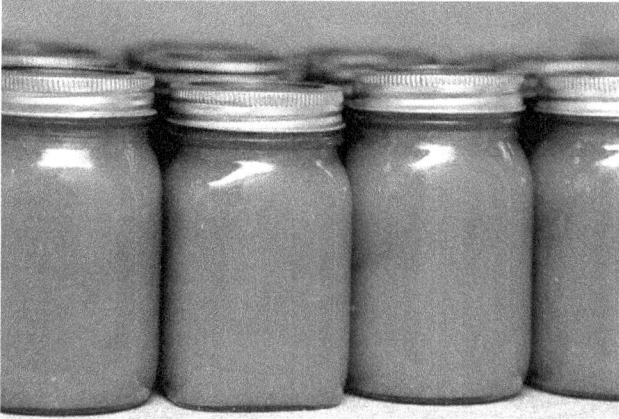

Recipe ID card

~ 17 Kcal calories per serving
~ Difficulty quite easy
~ Serves 10 people
~ Preparation 60 minutes
~ Low cost
~ About 60 minutes + the time needed to sterilize the jars

Ingredients

~ 2 Kg of San Marzano tomatoes
~ Optional: a few basil leaves

Material Required

~ Capacious bowls
~ Large casseroles
~ Tomato sauce machine or vegetable mill
~ Glass jars with respective screw caps
~ Tea towels
~ Tongs
~ Ladles of various sizes
~ Funnel
~ Pasta drainer

Preparation

Fill a large saucepan with water and turn on the heat until it comes to a boil.

In the meantime, wash the ripe tomatoes well in fresh water, then plunge them into the boiling water for about 5 minutes. The tomatoes can be removed from the water as soon as the skin breaks.

Let the tomatoes drain and cool in a colander.

In the meantime, sterilize the glass jars: immerse the jars (with their respective caps) in cold water, then bring to a boil.

Remove the skin from the tomatoes: the operation is very simple and can be done by hand.

Operate the tomato puree machine: collect the skins and scraps in a container, and the pulp in another. Alternatively, cut the tomatoes into pieces and mash them with a vegetable masher.

Inevitably, a very liquid tomato puree will be obtained because tomatoes contain a high quantity of water. In order to make the puree thicker, it is advisable to filter everything through a clean cloth, placed over a colander and a bowl. In the bowl will be collected the simple liquid, whereas in the dishcloth will be trapped the (thick) pulp of tomato.

Remove the jars from the water and fill them with the (raw) tomato puree. Those who wish can add a few basil leaves to the jars. Close with the screw cap and sterilize the jars with the passata.

Store jars of tomato puree in a cool, dry place for up to one year.

Wholewheat Brisé Pasta

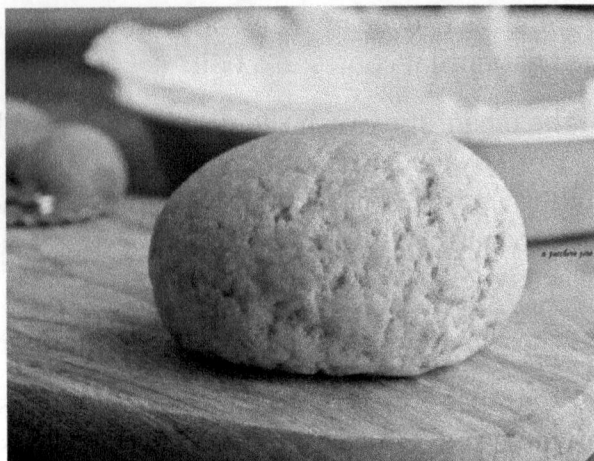

Preparation

Combine whole wheat flour in a bowl. Combine sifted instant yeast and salt. Stir in dry ingredients.

In the center, add the natural soy yogurt, extra virgin olive oil (or seed oil) and water. Knead all ingredients, first with a wooden spoon, then by hand until a soft dough is obtained.

Wrap the dough in a sheet of plastic wrap and let it rest for half an hour: in this way, it will be easier to roll out.

Roll out the dough with a rolling pin until the desired thickness is obtained. Use as desired to create appetizers or pies.

Recipe ID card

~ 329 Kcal calories per serving
~ Difficulty very easy
~ Serves 8
~ Preparation 15 minutes
~ Low cost
~ 15 minutes + 30 minutes for resting

Ingredients

~ 225 g of wholemeal flour
~ 75 g of soy yogurt
~ 45 ml of extra virgin olive oil
~ 30 ml of water
~ 6 g of salt
~ Half a teaspoon of instant yeast

Material Required

~ Bowl
~ Wooden spoon
~ Transparent film
~ Food scale
~ Rolling pin

Pesto Genovese style

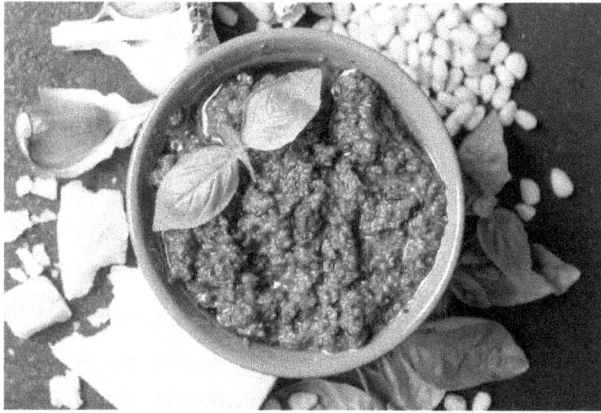

Recipe ID card

~ 492 Kcal calories per serving
~ Difficulty fairly easy
~ Serves 6
~ Preparation 20 minutes
~ Low cost
~ 20 minutes + time for cleaning and drying basil

Ingredients

~ 40 g of basil leaves
~ 30 g of pine nuts
~ 25 g of grated grana cheese
~ 25 g of pecorino cheese
~ (about 50-60 ml) of extra virgin olive oil
~ coarse salt
~ 1 clove of garlic

Material Required

~ Marble mortar and pestle
~ Grater
~ Glass jars for storage
~ Frying pan for toasting pine nuts
~ Spoons
~ Blotting paper or soft cloths to dry the basil

Preparation

Gently wash the basil leaves and dry them with a soft cloth or paper towels.

Remove the heart from the garlic clove: in this way, the pesto will be more digestible.

Pour the garlic clove and a few grains of coarse salt into a mortar, then begin to crush with the pestle until a cream is obtained.

Toast the pine nuts in a pan, without adding oil or other seasonings. In this way, the aroma of the pine nuts will be better released.

Add the basil leaves a few at a time and cover with more coarse salt grains: with gentle rotating movements, pound the leaves until they form a cream.

Now add the pine nuts and continue to pound with the pestle.

Once a cream is obtained, add the grated grana cheese, the grated pecorino cheese and enough extra virgin olive oil to obtain the desired consistency.

The pesto is ready to be stored in sterilized glass jars, well covered with a little oil to avoid the formation of mold.

Rocket Pesto

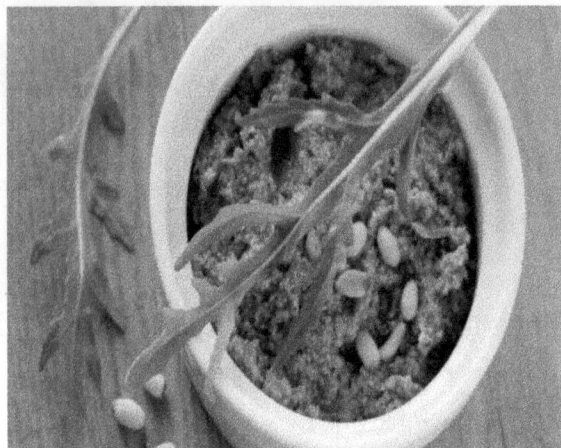

Recipe ID card

~ 362 Kcal calories per serving
~ Easy difficulty
~ Serves 6
~ Preparation 15 minutes
~ Low cost

Ingredients

~ 80 g of rocket
~ 50 g of grated Parmesan cheese
~ 30 g of pine nuts
~ 50 g of pecorino cheese
~ salt
~ 3 spoons of water
~ 2 tablespoons of extra virgin olive oil

Material Required

~ Mortar and pestle
~ Bowl
~ Frying pan
~ Blender
~ Grater

Preparation

Wash and dry the arugula.

Toast the pine nuts to bring out their aroma. Heat a frying pan and add the pine nuts: keep a moderate flame and stir often to avoid burning them. The pine nuts are ready when they give off an intense aroma. Leave to cool.

Blend the pecorino cheese and grate the grana cheese.

Pour one part of the pine nuts into a mortar, add one part of the arugula and grind everything with a pestle. Continue in this way, a little at a time, until all the arugula has been used up.

Now mix the arugula and pine nut pesto with the two grated cheeses and the salt. Mix everything with a few tablespoons of oil and water.

Keep in the fridge, covering with extra virgin olive oil and consume within 5 days.

LIGHT Meat Sauce

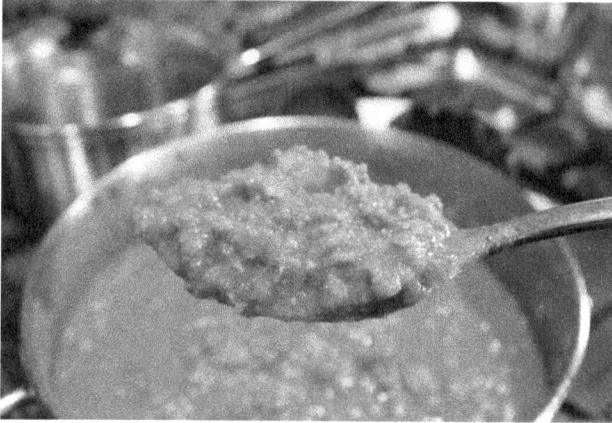

Recipe ID card

- ~ 78 Kcal calories per serving
- ~ Easy difficulty
- ~ Serves 4
- ~ Preparation 110 minutes
- ~ Average cost
- ~ 20 minutes for preparation; 90 minutes for cooking

Ingredients

- ~ 350 g of mixed lean ground meat
- ~ pepper
- ~ salt
- ~ 1-2 celery stalks
- ~ 1 garlic clove
- ~ 100 g (1 medium) carrots
- ~ 1 grated nutmeg
- ~ 1 pinch of cinnamon
- ~ 1 bay leaf
- ~ A few leaves of sage
- ~ 1 sprig of rosemary
- ~ 1 tablespoon of tomato paste
- ~ 200 ml (about 1 glass) of dry white wine

Material Required

- ~ Casserole dish with lid
- ~ Sterile gauze
- ~ Wooden spoon
- ~ Vegetable peeler
- ~ Knife
- ~ Blender

Preparation

Clean the vegetables, then peel the carrot and wash it thoroughly. Wash celery. Cut carrot and celery into pieces, then obtain a fine chop with the help of an electric blender.

Prepare the aromas: in a sterile gauze combine the sage, rosemary, bay leaf and garlic clove. Weld the end of the gauze with a kitchen string.

Brown the minced meat in a very hot saucepan, taking care to deglaze the mince with a wooden spoon and maintain a high flame.

Add the tomato paste (or the tomato puree), the chopped vegetables and the aromatic gauze to the minced meat, which in the meantime will be perfectly browned. If you wish, you can also add a shallot.

Season with salt and pepper and add spices such as cinnamon and nutmeg. Cover the minced meat with white wine (or red wine) and bring to boil.

Once it comes to the boil, lower the heat and cook over very low heat for about 1 hour and a half, until the liquid has partially dried up.

It is advisable to check often the cooking and, if necessary, add more liquid.

Vegan Ricotta Cheese - Soy Cheese

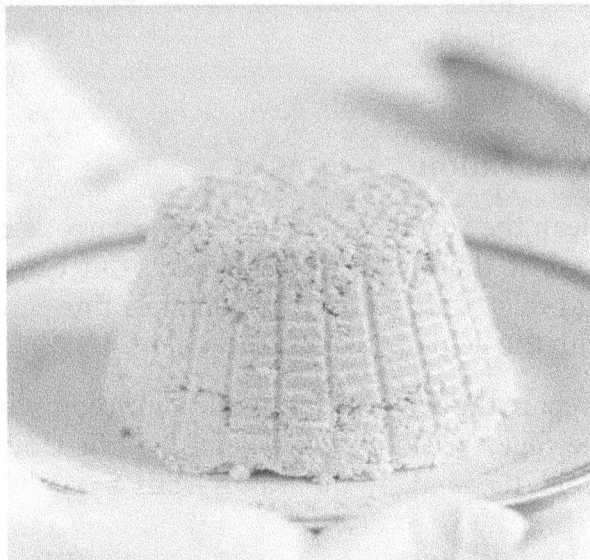

Recipe ID card

~ Difficulty quite easy
~ Serves 4
~ Preparation 110 minutes
~ Low cost
~ 20 minutes for preparation; 90 minutes for draining

Ingredients

~ 1 L of soy milk
~ 30 ml apple vinegar or 30 ml untreated lemon juice
~ salt

Material Required

~ Casserole
~ Wooden ladle
~ Large bowl
~ Cloth
~ Pasta strainer
~ Bundle
~ Saucer
~ Transparent film

Preparation

Pour unsweetened soy milk (preferably homemade) into a small saucepan and bring almost to a boil, maintaining a moderate flame.

Pour the hot soy milk into a glass bowl and add the apple cider vinegar. Stir for one minute. Cover with a sheet of plastic wrap and let stand 10 minutes.

After 10 minutes, the curd will have formed, so you can proceed with filtration (i.e., separating the whey from the vegetable ricotta). Line a colander with a cotton cloth that does not smell of detergent. Then place the colander over a narrow, large bowl. Pour the curdled soy milk into the colander lined with the dishcloth and let it drain for about an hour and a half, stirring occasionally to facilitate the operation.

Once most of the whey has been separated from the veg-cheese, salt to taste by stirring the thick curd with a wooden spoon. In this phase it is possible to flavor the ricotta with spices and aromas such as parsley, basil, paprika etc..

Remove the vegetable ricotta from the cloth and transfer it to a cheese mould: in this way, the cheese will take the precise shape of a ricotta.

If necessary, allow the ricotta to drain (in the cheese pan) to remove excess whey.

Store vegetable ricotta in the refrigerator and consume within 2-3 days.

Citronette Sauce and Vinaigrette Sauce

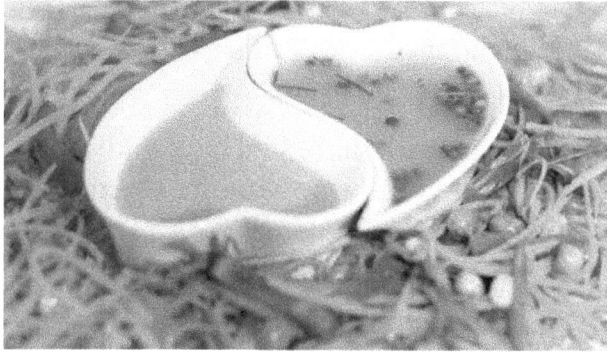

Recipe ID card

- ~ 545 Kcal calories per serving
- ~ Difficulty very easy
- ~ Serves 8
- ~ Preparation 10 minutes
- ~ Low cost

Ingredients

For the citronette sauce

- ~ 3 tablespoons of extra virgin olive oil
- ~ Untreated lemon juice and zest
- ~ 1 tablespoon pink pepper
- ~ A few stems of chives
- ~ Salt

For the vinaigrette sauce (French Dressing)

- ~ pepper
- ~ salt
- ~ 2 tablespoons vinegar
- ~ 3 tablespoons extra virgin olive oil
- ~ 1 teaspoon of mustard

Material Required

- ~ Glass jar
- ~ Immersion mixer (optional)
- ~ Bowls

Preparation

Preparation of Citronette Sauce. In a glass jar, pour the oil, lemon juice, chopped chives, salt and pink peppercorns. Close the jar with a screw top and shake well. Pour into a small bowl and use as desired.

Preparing the Vinaigrette Sauce. Combine the white wine vinegar, oil, salt, pepper and mustard paste in a beaker. Emulsify everything with an immersion blender. Pour into a bowl and serve to taste.

Cren Sauce

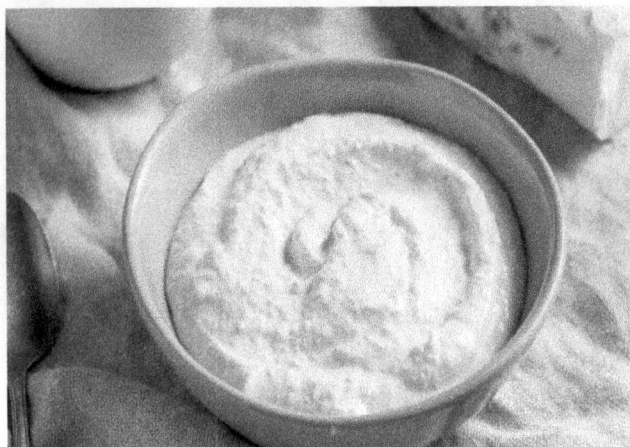

Cut the root into small pieces, then combine in a blender. Chop the horseradish until the mixture is not too coarse.

Mix the chopped horseradish with a pinch of salt and a teaspoon of sugar.

Fill glass jars with the grated horseradish pulp, then add enough wine vinegar to cover the surface.

Store in the refrigerator. It is recommended to wait at least one month before consumption.

Recipe ID card

~ Easy difficulty
~ Serves 10 people
~ Preparation 15 minutes
~ Low cost

Ingredients

~ 100 g of horseradish root
~ about 100 ml vinegar
~ salt
~ 1 teaspoon of sugar

Material Required

~ Grater or electric blender
~ Glass jars with screw cap
~ Vegetable peeler
~ Knife
~ Bowls

Preparation

Wash and brush the horseradish root. Remove the rind with a knife or vegetable peeler.

Tuna sauce LIGHT

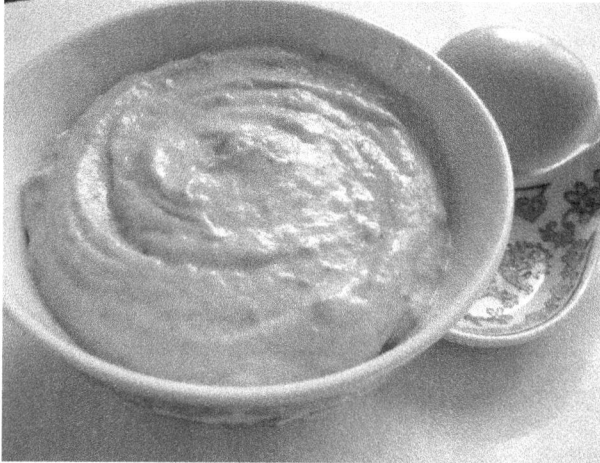

Mix everything for a couple of minutes, until the tuna becomes a cream. To facilitate the operation, pour into the mixer a few teaspoons of Greek yogurt.

Mix the cream obtained with the remaining Greek yogurt (0% fat). Adjust salt if necessary.

The sauce is ready to accompany meat and fish or simply to prepare irresistible canapés.

Recipe ID card

~ 134 Kcal calories per serving
~ Difficulty very easy
~ Serves 8
~ Preparation 10 minutes
~ Low cost

Ingredients

~ 150 g of drained tuna in oil
~ 150 g of Greek yogurt
~ 30 g of capers
~ 2 anchovy fillets

Material Required

~ Electric blender
~ Bowls
~ Spoons
~ Knives

Preparation

Drain well the tuna in oil and pour into a blender. Add the capers and anchovies.

Homemade Sesame Sauce

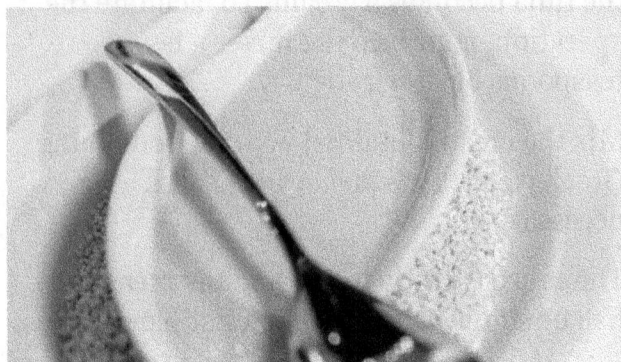

Recipe ID card

~ 650 Kcal calories per serving
~ Easy difficulty
~ Serves 8
~ Preparation 15 minutes
~ Average cost

Ingredients

~ 100 g of sesame seeds
~ 30 ml of sesame seed oil or grape seed oil
~ 1 pinch of salt

Material Required

~ Blender or mortar
~ Stone or non-stick frying pan
~ Gravy boat
~ Small bowl
~ Wooden spoon

Preparation

Spread the sesame seeds in a pan and toast them for a few minutes, keeping the flame very gentle. During toasting it is recommended to continuously stir sesame seeds in order to prevent them from darkening, developing bitter compounds and potentially dangerous for the health. However toasting is a very important operation in order to exalt the aroma of tahina. As an alternative, toast sesame seeds in the oven for 5-6 minutes, at a temperature of 180°C (350°F).

Pour the sesame seeds into a blender, add 3 tablespoons of grape seed oil (or sesame seed oil), add salt to taste and run the blender.

The sauce is ready when the sesame seeds are perfectly blended.

Allow the sauce to cool and serve on croutons. The tahina sauce can be stored in properly sterilized glass jars.

Example Diet

<u>Retired lady who is able to take long walks. She takes hypoglycemic medications.</u>

Sex F

Age 77

Height 155 cm

Wrist circumference 15.5 cm

Constitution Normal

Height/wrist 10.0

Morphological type Normal

Weight kg 68

Body Mass Index 28.3

Assessment Overweight

Desirable physiological body mass index 21.7

Desirable Physiologic Weight kg   52,1

Basal metabolic rate kcal 1134.6

Physical activity level coefficient SI aus 1.56

Energy expenditure kcal 1769.9

Hypochaloric Diet -30% 1240 Kcal about

Lipids 30% 372kcal 41.3g

Protein 1.2g/kg * physiol. weight 250.1kcal 62.5g

Carbohydrates 50.0% 617.9kcal 164.8g

Breakfast 15% 186kcal

Snack 10% 124kcal

Lunch 35% 434kcal

Snack 10% 124kcal

Dinner 30% 372kcal

Note. The example diet that follows refers to a case of diabetes mellitus type 2 already pharmacologically compensated; therefore, the use of pasta and bread is allowed; however, even if glycemia would be higher, it would not be possible to excessively distort the nutritional balance of the diet in favor of fats (which would limit weight loss) and/or proteins (which could excessively fatigue the liver and kidneys of a subject in old age).

Example diet for Diabetes Type 2

DAY 1

Breakfast,	about 15%kcal TOT
Low-fat milk,	2% of total 150ml, 75.0kcal
Wholemeal bread, stale bread.	50g, 121,5kcal
Snack,	about 10%kcal TOT
Low-fat yogurt	125g, 70,0kcal
Strawberries	150g, 48,0kcal
Lunch,	about 35%kcal TOT
Pasta with tomato sauce	
Whole wheat pasta	80g, 259,2kcal
Tomato sauce	100g, 24,0kcal
Parmesan cheese	10g, 39,2kcal
Lettuce	100g, 18.0kcal
Extra virgin olive oil	15g, 135,0kcal
Snack,	about 10%kcal TOT
Low-fat yogurt	125g, 70,0kcal
Sour red cherries	100g, 50,0kcal
Dinner,	about 30%kcal TOT
Grilled chicken breast	
Chicken breast	100g, 110,0kcal
Eggplant	200g, 48,0kcal
Wholemeal bread	25g, 60,8kcal
Extra virgin olive oil	15g, 135.0kcal

DAY 2

Breakfast,	about 15%kcal TOT
Low-fat milk,	2% of total 150ml, 75.0kcal
Wholemeal bread, stale bread	50g, 121,5kcal
Snack,	about 10% kcal TOT
Low-fat yogurt	125g, 70,0kcal
½ orange	200g, 63,0kcal
Lunch,	about 35%kcal TOT
Stewed beans	
Dried beans	80g, 279,9kcal
Parmesan cheese	10g, 39,2kcal
Radicchio	100g, 24,0kcal
Extra virgin olive oil	15g, 135,0kcal
Snack,	about 10%kcal TOT
Low-fat yogurt	125g, 70,0kcal
½ orange	200g, 63,0kcal
Dinner,	about 30%kcal TOT
Trout fillet	
Trout, various species	100g, 148,0kcal
Fennel	200g, 62,0kcal
Wholemeal bread	25g, 60,8kcal
Extra virgin olive oil	10g, 90.0kcal

DAY 3

Breakfast,	about 15%kcal TOT
Low-fat milk,	2% of total 150ml, 75.0kcal
Wholemeal bread, stale bread	50g, 121,5kcal
Snack,	about 10%kcal TOT
Low-fat yogurt	125g, 70,0kcal
½ apple, with peel	200g, 52,0kcal
Lunch,	about 35%kcal TOT
Plain rice	
Brown rice	80g, 289,6kcal
Parmesan cheese	10g, 39,2kcal
Arugula	100g, 25,0kcal
Extra virgin olive oil	15g, 135,0kcal
Snack,	about 10%kcal TOT
Low-fat yogurt	125g, 70,0kcal
½ apple, with peel	200g, 52,0kcal
Dinner,	about 30%kcal TOT
Hard-boiled eggs	
Chicken grape	100g, 143,0kcal
Potato	100g, 85,0kcal
Wholemeal bread	25g, 60.8kcal
Extra virgin olive oil	5g, 45.0kcal

DAY 4

Breakfast,	about 15%kcal TOT
Low-fat milk,	2% of total 150ml, 75.0kcal
Wholemeal bread, stale bread	50g, 121,5kcal
Snack,	about 10%kcal TOT
Low-fat yogurt	125g, 70,0kcal
Kiwi	100g, 61,0kcal
Lunch,	about 35%kcal TOT
Chickpeas in broth	
Chickpeas, dried	90g, 300,6kcal
Parmesan cheese	10g, 39,2kcal
Valerian	100g, 18,0kcal
Extra virgin olive oil	15g, 135,0kcal
Snack,	about 10%kcal TOT
Low-fat yogurt	125g, 70,0kcal
Kiwi	100g, 61,0kcal
Dinner,	about 30%kcal TOT
Pan-fried cod fillet	
Atlantic cod fillet	100g, 82,0kcal
Swiss chard	200g, 38,0kcal
Whole wheat bread	25g, 60,8kcal
Extra virgin olive oil	15g, 135,0kcal

DAY 5

Breakfast,	about 15%kcal TOT
Low-fat milk,	2% of total 150ml, 75.0kcal
Wholemeal bread, stale bread	50g, 121,5kcal
Snack,	about 10%kcal TOT
Low-fat yogurt	125g, 70,0kcal
Strawberries	150g, 48,0kcal
Lunch,	about 35%kcal TOT
Eggplant pasta	
Whole wheat pasta	80g, 259,2kcal
Eggplant	100g, 24,0kcal
Parmesan cheese	10g, 39,2kcal
Lettuce	100g, 18.0kcal
Extra virgin olive oil	15g, 135,0kcal
Snack,	about 10%kcal TOT
Low-fat yogurt	125g, 70,0kcal
Sour red cherries	100g, 50,0kcal
Dinner,	about 30%kcal TOT
Turkey breast	
Chicken breast	100g, 111,0kcal
Zucchini	200g, 36,0kcal
Wholemeal bread	25g, 60,8kcal
Extra virgin olive oil	15g, 135.0kcal

DAY 6

Breakfast,	about 15%kcal TOT
Low-fat milk,	2% of total 150ml, 75.0kcal
Wholemeal bread, stale bread	50g, 121,5kcal
Snack,	about 10%kcal TOT
Low-fat yogurt	125g, 70,0kcal
½ orange	200g, 63,0kcal
Lunch,	about 35%kcal TOT
Stewed beans	
Dried beans	80g, 279,9kcal
Parmesan cheese	10g, 39,2kcal
Radicchio	100g, 24,0kcal
Extra virgin olive oil	15g, 135,0kcal
Snack,	about 10%kcal TOT
Low-fat yogurt	125g, 70,0kcal
½ orange	200g, 63,0kcal
Dinner,	about 30%kcal TOT
Trout fillet	
Trout, various species	100g, 97,0kcal
Fennel	200g, 62,0kcal
Wholemeal bread	25g, 60,8kcal
Extra virgin olive oil	15g, 135,0kcal

DAY 7

Breakfast,	about 15%kcal TOT
Low-fat milk,	2% of total 150ml, 75.0kcal
Wholemeal bread, stale bread	50g, 121,5kcal
Snack,	about 10%kcal TOT
Low-fat yogurt	125g, 70,0kcal
½ apple, with peel	200g, 52,0kcal
Lunch,	about 35%kcal TOT
Plain rice	
Brown rice	80g, 289,6kcal
Parmesan cheese	10g, 39,2kcal
Arugula	100g, 25,0kcal
Extra virgin olive oil	15g, 135,0kcal
Snack,	about 10%kcal TOT
Low-fat yogurt	125g, 70,0kcal
½ apple, with peel	200g, 52,0kcal
Dinner,	about 30%kcal TOT
Ricotta cheese	
Cow's milk ricotta, partially skimmed	100g, 138,0kcal
Endive	200g, 36,0kcal
Wholemeal bread	25g, 60,8kcal
Extra virgin olive oil	10g, 90,0kcal

APPENDIX

Cooking Conversion Charts

INGREDIENTS	CONVERSION US	CONVERSION EU
cup	16 tablespoons	236 ml
fluid ounce – fl.oz.	–	30 ml
pinch / dash	1/16 teaspoon	–
pint	2 cups	0,47 l
pound	16 ounces	454 g
quart	4 cups	0,95 l
teaspoon – tsp	1/3 tablespoon	5 ml
tablespoon – tbsp	3 teaspoons	15 ml
ounce – oz	–	28 g

Dry Ingredients

INGREDIENTS	CONVERSION
Cake/Pastry Flour	1 cup : 115 g
All-purpose	1 cup : 125 g
High gluten	1 cup : 140 g
Whole wheat	1 cup : 120 g
Bread flour	1 cup : 130 g
Spelt	1 cup : 100 g
Light Rye	1 cup : 100 g
Dark Rye	1 cup : 125 g
Buckweat	1 cup : 120 g
Rice	1 cup : 185 g
Sugar	1 cup : 200 g
Brown Sugar	1 cup : 220 g
Powdered Sugar	1 cup : 120 g
Baking Soda	1 tsp : 5 g
Baking Powder	1 tsp : 5 g
Fresh yeast	1 tsp : 3 g
Active dry yeast	1 tsp : 3 g
Salt	1 tbsp : 18 g
Chocolate chips	1 cup : 160 g
Cocoa	1 cup : 120 g

Fresh ingredients

INGREDIENTS	CONVERSIONS
Water	1 cup : 236 ml
Milk	1 cup : 245 ml
Yogurt	1 cup : 245 ml
Cream	1 cup : 245 ml
Buttermilk	1 cup : 245 ml
Olive Oil	• 1 cup : 222 ml • 1 tbsp : 13 g
Butter	• 1 cup : 230 g • 1 tbsp : 14.5 g • 1 stick : 1/2 cup : 8 tbsp : 115 g
Eggs	1 cup : 275 g
(Egg) Whites	1 cup : 240 g
(Egg) Yolks	1 cup : 300 g
Honey	• 1 cup : 340 g • 1 tbsp : 20 g
Grated cheese	1 cup : 110 g
Vanilla extract	1 tsp : 4 g
Peanut Butter	1 cup : 258 g

Oven Temperatures

250 °F	120 °C
275 °F	140 °C
300 °F	150 °C
325 °F	160 °C
350 °F	180 °C
375 °F	190 °C
400 °F	200 °C
425 °F	220 °C
450 °F	230 °C
475 °F	240 °C
500 °F	260 °C

www.ingramcontent.com/pod-product-compliance
Lightning Source LLC
Chambersburg PA
CBHW080627030426
42336CB00018B/3102